Dedicated to my patients - past, present, and future - who courageously step forward in pursuit of the dream of motherhood (and fatherhood), and to my beautiful adopted children who showed me that love truly transcends all.

"Your own positive future begins in this moment.
All you have is right now. Every goal is possible from here."
- Lao Tzu

Printed in the United States of America

First Printing, 2019

ISBN 978-1-7323017-1-9

Axelrad Clinic, LLC
19 Briar Hollow Lane, Suite 240
Houston, TX 77027

www.axelradclinic.com
frontdesk@axelradclinic.com

"Chris is one of the most compassionate and educated practitioners in his chosen field of acupuncture and Chinese medicine, and especially when it comes to treating women struggling with infertility. He understands his patient's truest desires and helps them to slow down, breathe, tap into, and listen to their own inner wisdom to achieve the outcome they desire."
- Melissa Cram, Acupuncture Physician, FL

"First off, he cares. He really really cares. And he'll give you hope, and help you heal yourself so anything is possible."
- Katy Szabo, Acupuncturist

"He helped me so much with getting my depression under control and body back in balance after several miscarriages so I could have my second child."
- Islin Munisteri – Author and Speaker

"I went to one of the "top" fertility guys in Houston when I was 40 and wanted to conceive. He told me I had a 3% chance of getting pregnant. My mother, grandmother and two sisters had already had cancer and it was estrogen positive cancer. IVF and other hormone treatments simply weren't an option for me. Within 3 months after seeing Chris, I was pregnant. I followed his advice to the letter - from doing the treatments to making dietary changes. I ncvcr fclt better in my entire life. Looking at my middle-school aged daughter now, I'm grateful I went to him."
- Molly Q (Chris' first fertility patient ever 😊)

"I have personally met this guy and know his intentions are to help people. His knowledge of both eastern and western sciences allow him to see things from both perspectives. But ultimately his ability to truly want happiness for all kinds is what is key."
- Jamie Catlett, Acupuncture Physician

"Chris is a professional with high integrity. He is open, honest and generously shares his experience and extensive knowledge."
  - Gabby Clark

"Chris actually cares. If you ever had a chance to speak with him in person, you will find out quickly that he emanates peace like no other person you've probably met. That's the kind of people I need around me. Reading this book has gone a long way towards helping me understanding how he does what he does."
  - David Roger Thompson

"Chris has a unique ability to be 100% forcefully honest and 100% compassionately kind. His advice is solid, clinical skills exceptional, and provides patients with solutions to real problems."
  - Janet L Borges, L.Ac.

"Yo le diría que aparte de ser una buen ser humano es un exelente Doctor el cual me ayudo para poder quedar embarazada y con su ayuda tube mis 3 hijos"
(I'm telling you that apart from being a good person, he's an excellent doctor because he helped me to stay pregnant after many miscarriages and with his help I now have 3 children.)
  - Yessenia M.

"Chris pours his heart and soul into helping others. His true passion is to help people heal and see them succeed in life. His advice is backed by science, studies, and years of personal experience in his practice."
  - Malorie Nicole, Transformational Coach

TABLE OF CONTENTS

Part One - Reclaiming Your Power

Part Two - Core Daily Rituals For Optimal Egg Quality

Part Three - Amplifying The Signal With Targeted Supplements

Part Four - Keeping Your Focus

Appendix

Disclaimer

This book details the author's clinical experience with and opinions about fertility enhancement and egg quality optimization. The author is not your healthcare provider.

The author and publisher are providing this book and its contents on an "as is" basis and make no representations or warranties of any kind with respect to this book or its contents. The author and publisher disclaim all such representations and warranties, including for example warranties of merchantability and healthcare for a particular purpose. In addition, the author and publisher do not represent or warrant that the information accessible via this book will lead to any specific result for the reader.

The statements made about products and services have not been evaluated by the U.S. Food and Drug Administration. They are not intended to diagnose, treat, cure, or prevent any condition or disease. Please consult with your own physician or healthcare specialist regarding the suggestions and recommendations made in this book.

Neither the author or publisher, contributors, or other representatives will be liable for damages arising out of or in connection with the use of this book.

You understand that this book is not intended as a substitute for consultation with a licensed healthcare practitioner, such as your physician. Before you begin any healthcare program or change your lifestyle in any way, you are responsible for consulting your physician or another licensed healthcare practitioner to ensure that the examples contained in this book will not harm you.

Use of this book implies acceptance of all terms stated within this disclaimer.

Something Important To Keep In Mind As You're Reading This Book

Yes, we have treatment options for people outside the Houston area to help you optimize your egg quality and get pregnant as soon as possible.

Visit https://axelradclinic.com/remote for details and availability.

AND

Because you're reading this book, **you have FREE, lifetime access to the Axelrad Clinic Academy,** our exclusive patient reference library that contains all the resources mentioned in this book and more, including:

- Simplified meal plans.
- Meditations and guided visualization tracks.
- Exclusive cheat sheets and critical reference materials.
- A special supportive online community of others who have or are still walking the same journey as you.
- Videos and other exclusive content only available to

Sign up for free, no strings attached, at
https://axelradclinic.com/awaken.

Acknowledgements

This book would not be possible without the support of so many amazing people who have been part of my life journey.

Obviously, first and foremost, my parents who instilled in me a powerful work ethic and a strong sense of purpose.

Secondly, my wife and children who have been my rock and support over the past 15 years as I built my practice.

To my most precious mentors including:
- The late Dr. Ray Rubio, the driving force behind the creation and early formation of The American Board of Oriental Reproductive Medicine (ABORM), who took me under his wing and taught me to believe in my leadership abilities.
- Dr. Randine Lewis, author of *The Infertility Cure*, who graciously trained and taught many of the "2nd generation" fertility acupuncturists here in the states, before specialized training resources were as widely available as there are today.
- Dr. Jerry Allan Johnson, a true pioneer and legend in the field of Medical Qigong. His training was pivotal in much of what you are going to read in this book.
- The physicians and staff of *Houston Fertility Institute* (https://www.hfi-ivf.com) who have entrusted me with caring for over a thousand of their patients during IVF, and who have been great mentors and friends on many levels.

And, of course, to all my amazing patients. They are the ones who inspire me every day to do my best. So much gratitude for them and the blessing of working with them every single day.

Chris Axelrad, M.S.O.M., L.Ac., FABORM, Houston, TX - 2018

Patient Testimonials

Quick note: All these patients have given birth to healthy babies. I tell you this only because in some cases the testimonial was taken (with permission, of course) from an email during early pregnancy. :-)

(Names are changed for privacy purposes. Other than that, these are unedited.)

"I am a forty-year-old woman, who is a newlywed of six months. One of my shared goals with my husband was to try to have a baby of our own. Honestly, at my age, I truly did not believe it was possible, but I was more than willing to try every natural resource before giving up. My husband and I decided to go to a fertility doctor and get a full workup on both of us. This way we would know if it was still possible for either one of us to conceive. This takes a good 6-8 weeks to get all the tests done. At the same time, I decided to get the name of an acupuncturist. A doctor friend of mine who was undergoing breast cancer treatments and seeing Chris to combat the effects of the chemo recommended him. I had never had acupuncture before. After my first meeting with Chris, he recommended a diet change. I wanted to lose about 15 pounds before I got pregnant. I was suffering from poor circulation, bad nutrition, and low energy. I followed Chris' instructions to the letter. I lost six pounds the first week and detoxed the heck out of my body. I started feeling so much better. In fact, I said to my husband one day, "I had no idea I could ever feel this good again. If I had, I would have made the necessary changes years ago." After only four sessions with Chris, I was pregnant. That entire month, I followed a healthy diet, exercised, took the vitamins he recommended, took the herbs he recommended and relaxed. Before I got pregnant, I lost a total of 13 pounds. The irony here is that the fertility doctor I went to said I could not get pregnant without insemination. I'm now 5 weeks pregnant and feeling really good. I

continue to see Chris and will continue throughout my pregnancy. I cannot tell enough people that this is how I got pregnant. There is absolutely no doubt in my mind. I have enjoyed this experience so much that my stepson and husband are now in the process of seeing Chris. I now believe there is so much more to learn about health and the body. I look forward to the growth I am experiencing and the guidance I receive from Chris."

"I am so grateful I came to visit Chris and give acupuncture a try. My husband and I had been trying to start a family for nine months and did not seem to have any luck. My menstrual cycles were exceptionally long and painful. I also was under a great deal of stress at my job. Chris was a great listener and very helpful to me in numerous ways. Acupuncture combined with herbal medicine helped me feel better physically and mentally. I felt more relaxed and was able to think more clearly. I also experienced less pains during my menstrual cycle. Most importantly, the acupuncture and medicine helped the length of my menstrual cycle decrease. These changes as a result of therapy, I believe enabled me to achieve my goal of starting a family. After four months of working with Chris, I became pregnant and am now expecting a little girl in less than 6 weeks!! I highly recommend trying acupuncture and/or herbal medicine with Chris if you are experiencing any stress, depression, having problems with your menstrual cycle, or having difficulty becoming pregnant. This experience has been a huge blessing in my life."

"My husband and I had been trying to conceive for nearly 18 months. Because I was older than 35, my OB-GYN wanted us to begin testing for possible infertility after six months, but we spread it out a little bit longer. After completing blood tests, HSG and semen analysis, nothing indicated why we had not been successful. We decided to do IUI as this was the most "natural" form of insemination. The first

round was not successful, so we scheduled a second round for the next cycle. In the meantime, I decided to try acupuncture due to reading other testimonials about the successful outcomes at The Axelrad Clinic. I am not exactly sure how long I met with Chris, but I don't think it was more than an entire cycle before I got pregnant. We did that second IUI, but I honestly believe it was done too soon because I didn't actually ovulate until four days later (I misread my signs). I believe that the theory behind acupuncture, treating the whole body, is what was required to get my system in sync. I have recommended acupuncture to friends who have had trouble conceiving and they have also experienced success."

"I came to Chris for acupuncture treatments in November 2006, in preparation for my first IVF cycle in January 2007. Immediately, I was impressed by his approachable manner, knowledge of infertility, and his willingness to incorporate my needs and concerns into the overall treatment approach. Since the main reason why we were doing IVF was because of my husband's severe male factor infertility, the main focus of my treatments with Chris was to promote my general level of fertility, while bringing other systems into balance. We also worked with relaxation techniques and focused breathing, which allowed me to better deal with stressful situations. Unlike other acupuncturists I had met in the past, Chris focused on a few key areas to promote my fertility and increase our chances for IVF success, rather than "throwing everything but the kitchen sink at the problem," as he put it. I followed his easy and helpful dietary changes and came in for treatments once a week until the IVF cycle began, then two times during the ovarian stimulation phase and before the embryo transfer. Two weeks after the embryo transfer, we found out the first IVF cycle was a success! I am now pregnant with our first child, who is due October 16, 2007. There is no doubt in my mind that our successful IVF cycle is due in part to the acupuncture treatments and stress relief techniques from the Axelrad Clinic of Chinese Medicine. I

highly recommend him as a very knowledgeable acupuncturist who specializes in the realm of infertility, and who takes a personal interest in your determination to overcome infertility."

"My best friend got pregnant through the assistance of acupuncture after a struggling with infertility issues for 5 years. Now, she is a mother of two beautiful children.

"When my husband and I finally decided that it was time to start a family after seven years of marriage, we were very hopeful that we'd get pregnant immediately. After six months of trying to conceive naturally with no luck and constant attention to my cycle, I visited my OBGYN, who told me to wait one full year to pursue fertility treatments. I was not in the mindset to wait, so I pursued visiting a fertility specialist. After running lab work, an ultrasound and an HSG, she diagnosed me with PCOS (polycystic ovarian syndrome), insulin resistance and suggested that I try to lose some weight. She also had my husband's sperm tested, which also posed challenges for our conceiving naturally.

"Rather than start medical fertility treatments right away, I decided that maybe my friend had found the answer through acupuncture. I contacted The Axelrad Clinic and began working with Chris to help treat our fertility issues and the anxiety that I was feeling about the process. From the beginning, he was very thorough and detailed. He taught me ways to deal with my anxiety and to think about my fertility in a new light.

"After seeing Chris consistently for four months, I decided that it was time to pursue assisted reproductive therapy. We chose to do an IUI and hormone injections along with a round of acupuncture. I had done my homework and discovered that the success rate for IUI was only 20%, so I was not expecting a positive pregnancy result. Yet, two

weeks later, I actually did receive a positive result! I am confident that the lifestyle changes I had made (losing weight and eating healthier) along with the acupuncture and the IUI procedure resulted in conception. I just returned from my 8-week OBGYN appointment where I saw the baby's heart pumping.

"I am so very thankful to Chris Axelrad for his patience in working with me through some heartbreakingly difficult months, listening to me and for guiding me through the fertility process. If you are experiencing fertility issues, I highly encourage you to meet with Chris and let him give you a new perspective!"

"I thought I'd attach a pic of my son Benjamin, who was born 11/17/08. He was a healthy 9 lb. 7 oz and 21.5 inches long and is now almost 11 lbs and 24.5 inches. I am very glad I opted to work with you to ensure the best outcome with my IVF!"

"Hi Chris from the Women's Pavilion at Texas Children's. Went into labor on my own 1 day late. Ignored the contractions all day at work as I've had them for over a month that always dropped off to nothing. Once I got home, they didn't stop, and I could not sleep. Holy cow! This really was it! Our beautiful son graced us with his presence at nearly midnight on 8/26. He is alert and sweet and full of personality. we can't believe he is here. He is a great, calm baby, easy to console. He is also a big boy- 8lbs 6oz, 22.25" long. Thank you for all of your help in our journey. You were such an instrumental piece in keeping my sanity through IVF and beyond."

"Hello Chris, Just wanted to thank YOU for what you have done for us. We are pregnant!!! =) We truly believe that you were meant to be a part of the journey to our miracle and very grateful to have found

you. YOU are Awesome!!! We will keep you posted. Sincerely, Heather"

"Hi Chris and Caity, I received your warm letter and nice gift (baby on the go)! Thanks so much for being there for me at the most important moment in my life, expanding a family. The Axelrad Clinic truly has touched my life in ways beyond imagination and I am grateful for that. I want to wish you a Merry Christmas and blessed new year 2015! Suzy"

"Chris, I cancelled my appointment today before I got the news (bad time management). But I got a positive pregnancy test today!! I REALLY appreciate all your guidance and help with this!! I am so excited!! THANK THANK THANK YOU! Courtney"

"Dear Chris and Caity, I just received your package in the mail! (We moved the first of the year, so it was waiting at our old apartment for me). Thank you so much for the baby skin care sets- I can't wait to pamper our little guys with the products! I am so thankful for all of your care for me and the babies during my pregnancy and truly believe that your help along the way was a key factor in our being able to bring home 2 healthy baby boys. (And in helping me stay calm and relaxed during the entire process)! I hope to be able to bring the babies in to meet you all sometime soon! - Amy"

"I went to the doctor this morning because I broke out in hives from the progesterone injections. I've been putting cream on it and it's

gotten better but I wanted the doctor to look at it. While I was there he took blood and guess what? I'M PREGNANT!!!!!!!! I cannot thank you enough for all of your help. I won't see you this week because I'll be out of town, but I will see you the following week!! Thank you thank you thank you!!!! Regards, Tori"

"Hey Chris, Just wanted to let you know the retrieval went awesome! She got 20 eggs and of those, 18 fertilized! We'll have to wait 5 days to see how many of the 18 make it to blastocyst. I'll keep you posted. I have a business trip in Vegas next week, so I won't see you until the following week. Have a great rest of your weekend! - April"

"It's been awhile since I've seen you... Our little guy was born a little early via C-section on Mar 5th, a little underweight at 5lbs and 18 3/4in. He is growing and doing great. I can't thank you enough for everything you did for us."

"Hi Chris, How are you? Hope all is well at your end. I hope you remember me. I was the one with a history of unexplained miscarriages. Anyways, I just wanted to let you know that we have a healthy baby girl now :-) She is 11 months old now. We have named her Shreya. (In our parts, it means auspicious). Sorry for delayed email. (Blame it on procrastination :-D). I want to thank you for everything you did, and for helping us remain positive. Here is a pic of me and my daughter. :-) Regards, Amaya"

"I got a BFP yesterday!!! My husband and I are beyond excited. Thank you so much for your help. This has been such an amazing time in our lives - Sonya"

"Chris, I wanted to let y'all know that we saw two heartbeats today. They are 6 weeks and one day a long, so it is very early, but it was an incredible thing to see today after trying for 4 years. Thanks for your magical touch and I pray this will continue. - Scott"

"Hi Chris! It's been a while, hope all is well!! I wanted to share some exciting news with you since you have been a major part of this journey. We are pregnant!! What a blessing!! Back in April the doctor recommended, after 3 failed Clomid cycles, that we pursue IVF. In May I went to visit you and you gave me herbs to prepare me for IVF. I told you and my doctor that I would take the summer off and pursue IVF in the Fall. Well, to our big surprise, we conceived naturally, and I am 9 wks. pregnant today! We found out a couple of weeks ago and the doctor has been monitoring my pregnancy each week. Everything looks good, we have a strong heartbeat, baby is growing and developing, and we are praying for the best! I know it's still early, but I wanted to give you the news and thank you for all your help in getting me where we are today! :) I need to come and visit you and the staff soon!! All the best, Martha"

"Hello Chris, I'm really happy and excited to tell you that I'm pregnant. I will be meeting the doctor on Thursday for an ultrasound. My husband and I truly appreciate for all your support. God bless you. I will keep you posted. Thanks, Beth"

"Just wanted to send you a quick email, HCG is at 9300, progesterone at 30 (so they may increase the progesterone I'm taking just to be on the safe side), and estrogen looks great. We finally got to see something on ultrasound yesterday, not much but it's something! I

measured 5w1d which is spot on, follow up on Friday. I feel good other than breast tenderness which comes and goes in severity. Also, I'm not sleeping well the second half of the night, other than that things are moving right along!"

"Chris, hope you had a great weekend, ours was very successful! We retrieved 27 eggs on Friday and got a call on Saturday that we made 18 embryos! We are overjoyed with the great news and are feeling so very blessed. Thanks for all your help along the way. We are thinking we will transfer mid-April. See you soon! Thanks, Jill"

"Hope you're having a good day! Just wanted to let you know we heard two heartbeats this morning! We are so excited! Thank you so much for all of your support and guidance! See you Friday, Ellen"

"Hi Chris! Congrats on your new office! That is great. I also wanted to share some good news with you. I am pregnant! Thank you so much for all of your help. I will see you again next week. Sarah"

"Chris, I have some good news for you! We went in for our beta today and we are pregnant! Today I am 11 days post transfer and my beta came in at 745. I am so excited and grateful for good news after what has felt like a very long and rough road. Just wanted to let you know since you have been so supportive and helpful along the way. Hope you had a great trip! See you next week. Thanks, Julie"

"Hi Chris, I just wanted to share the wonderful news that I am now confirmed pregnant!!! Thank you for all the care you have given me during this journey. :) Xia"

"Hi Chris, I wanted to let you know I got my positive beta today at 307 (9 days post transfer!!) Finally :) Thanks for everything. Have a great 4th of July weekend. ~Katharine"

"Chris, I wanted to thank you for everything you've done and for all the times you listened to my silly worries. I will be back for more acupuncture, but for now we are saving up for our TWINS. Thank you thank you thank you. See you soon Chandra"

"Hi Chris, our daughter Lucia was born August 20th at 3:18 pm. She weighed 6 lbs 8 oz and is 19 inches long. We are so in love with her!! Thank you so much for everything you did for us to help us gain this precious gift! The comparison picture shows me on the left at the same age as Lucia on the right. We will be in touch soon! Sarah"

"Chris, it's been a while since I was a patient - my triplets will be 7 in January. I just wanted to drop you a quick note to say I look forward to Wednesdays to watch your short videos and hear your messages each week. I live in Austin now so can't pop by the clinic, but I wanted to take the time to say "thank you" for inspiring me each week to be a better person, wife and mother. Many thanks, Louisa"

"We are doing well... Ella Jane arrived on the 19th Oct (7lbs 9oz and 20.5") and the past month has been a blur!!! We are still getting used to her schedule (or lack thereof) and prioritizing sleep over anything other than her needs :) All is going well, and we are all in good

health. Thank you and please pass on my thanks to Chris, Jaime and Caity for their excellent help through my pregnancy! - Margaret"

"The Axelrad Clinic is amazing! From the moment you call, you are treated like family. They make setting appointments or rescheduling them a breeze. Chris was able to treat my anxiety, define an adrenal problem, and help with my overall health. I am a school teacher, and I used to get sick several times a year. Now I am healthy year-round! They recommend great brands of vitamins and even sell them online for refills! I first went to Chris for general health but am excited to begin working on fertility with him now as well! I recommend the clinic to all my family and friends and can't think of a better place to go to become healthy and whole!" - Jennifer

---

"I never thought I would face infertility. We were shocked and upset when IVF didn't work the first time. My doctor wanted to make sure I knew about all of my options and referred me to Chris for acupuncture. Chris really focused on my overall wellbeing. He addressed my stress (what stress?!), how well I was (not) sleeping and my (lack of) energy. Chris is highly knowledgeable and very easy to talk to. After all the needle pokes of IVF I wasn't too thrilled about more needles with acupuncture. That being said, you hardly feel them! It's now super relaxing and I usually doze off. I'm happy to say that we're now expecting our miracle baby! I'm so grateful for my entire medical team, including Chris and The Axelrad Clinic. I would definitely recommend The Axelrad Clinic to anyone struggling with infertility. The entire staff will make you feel right at home." - Kate

---

"When I went to see Chris, I had been struggling with infertility for two years. In that period, I had experienced an early miscarriage and two chemical pregnancies. A friend, who had also experienced

infertility and is now mother to a beautiful baby girl, highly recommended Chris. During my first appointment, Chris immediately put me at ease. He listened to my long history of infertility and took careful notes. He was reassuring and gave me such confidence. I left the appointment with a treatment plan that included recommended supplements, tips on nutrition and general recommendations to help me with my goal of getting pregnant. I was also hugely impressed with how they run the clinic. Everything is efficient and organized. At my second appointment with Chris, I told him that I was experiencing symptoms that I hadn't experienced since my first pregnancy and that I thought I might be pregnant. My fertility doctor confirmed my pregnancy the following day. I continued to see Chris weekly until I reached 12 weeks. I am now seeing them monthly until I reach 36 weeks, and then will see them weekly until I (hopefully!) deliver a healthy baby. As someone who has experienced pregnancy loss, those first 12 weeks were especially terrifying. I was so grateful for my weekly appointments with Chris. In those appointments, he patiently listened to my concerns and followed up on concerns I had expressed the previous week. I always left my appointments feeling relaxed and reassured. On one occasion, I came into my appointment extremely concerned with some cramping. I told Jaime (another clinician at The Axelrad Clinic) that I had a doctor's appointment in two days where we would have an ultrasound. I was so touched when I received an email in my inbox three days later, asking how my doctor's appointment went and checking to see if all was well. I am so very thankful to have Chris and his team as part of this journey and cannot recommend The Axelrad Clinic highly enough. This is a truly amazing team! - Tessa"

More testimonials, including videos, at
https://www.axelradclinic.com/success.

Why This Book Exists...

I grew up in a family of MDs. My father, all my uncles, a great uncle, and my brother are or were successful physicians.

My father - a now-retired surgeon - was a captain of a forward medical command in the Vietnam War. A 28-year old "man" at the time, who was at the time a newly minted surgeon fresh out of med school, he commanded the field hospital at an important 1st Cavalry Landing Zone in the heart of the South Vietnamese countryside, where he would tend to wounded and dying American soldiers and, as it turned out, countless Vietnamese civilians including children.

It was shortly after his return from the battlefield that he and my mother were married.

Soon afterwards, I was born. Not much later, when I was very young, they divorced.

As I'm sure many children of divorce do, I often wondered (even as a small child) if I had been a "mistake".

When I was 45 years old, I accompanied my father when he returned to Vietnam for the first time since the war, in search of an old friend he hadn't seen or heard from in all that time.

I got to witness firsthand the countryside where he was stationed. To say the least, I fully realized the unthinkable emotional impact that experience must have had on him.

That was ONE moment of closure for me in understanding why my parents had split up.

But, perhaps even more profound - at least in terms of how I ended up here writing this book - was the story my mother told me when, at 19 years old, I finally got up the courage to ask her what had happened between her and my father when I was little. I remember as part of that, I literally asked her the question…

"Mom, did you ever feel like I was a mistake?"

Her answer changed my life forever.

"In my late teens I was diagnosed with severe endometriosis," she said. "They told me I would never be able to have children because of it. So, I had accepted that and made peace with it.

"Then, I became pregnant with you. And it was like the greatest miracle ever. You were my miracle baby. There was never any question that you belonged here with me."

And, I realized that, indeed, I *wasn't* supposed to be here… according to what the doctors had told my mother (and she had accepted as fact).

Yet, here I was. Not a mistake. *A miracle.*

Fast-forward to around 2010, I'd been in practice as an acupuncturist for six years at that point - five of them as a specialist in fertility. I'd already helped several hundred patients overcome their fertility struggles at that point and wouldn't even have imagined that we'd help over 2000 more to do the same by early 2018.

Yet, to be honest, I never fully understood why I was so fascinated and inspired by the path I'd chosen as a fertility specialist.

As happens often, a patient and I were having a nice conversation as I was placing needles in her for treatment. Suddenly, she asks, "So, why did you decide to focus on fertility?"

Up until that point, nobody had asked me that. They'd routinely ask me why I got into Chinese Medicine when I came from an MD family. That was a question that popped up at least 2-3 times a month, if not more.

But, "Why did you decide to focus on fertility…?" Totally new question. I tried my best to give the most honest answer I could…

"My mom was told she couldn't have children and yet, here I am. So, my mission is to help other babies who 'aren't supposed to be here' to get here."

BAM. Like a lightning bolt. And, it all made sense from there.

I also realized upon further reflection that, indeed, my passion for women's health and gynecology - which preceded my journey into fertility as a specialty - was inspired by other aspects of my mother's story as well.

In so many ways, my mother is my hero and here are just a few reasons why:

1. The tremendous pain she suffered from endometriosis with no real treatment options at that time.
2. How she so courageously and skillfully raised my brother (from a later marriage) and I as a single mom.
3. Watching her start off as a teacher, then switch careers to become a successful real estate broker.
4. Then, after the real estate crash in Houston in the 80's, when she was 39 and I was in high-school, she enrolled in law

school, graduated at 42, and went on to become a legendary (and very successful) appellate attorney until she retired at 70 years old.

Took a lot of courage, focus, and determination to do all that. To say she overcame the odds in more ways than one would be a *massive* understatement.

So, my hope is this book serves as a turning point for you on *your* journey to becoming a mother - to beating the so-called "odds" and realizing *your* dream.

Because that mother-spirit inside you is one of the most powerful and special things we have in this human life.

And, while I can't promise you a baby, here's something I can promise:

This book, should you follow the action steps and put them into practice, will awaken and focus that mother-spirit like nothing else.

With Sincere Kindness and Gratitude,
Chris Axelrad, Houston, TX

Introduction

If you're having difficulty getting pregnant and you're looking for a proven, clear, and simple path so you can put an end to what I know can be an overwhelming and anxiety-provoking journey to start (or grow) your family… Rest assured, you're in the right place.

What you are about to encounter is, in my experience - and as you'll soon find out I've got a lot of experience - the simplest, most direct, most effective path for you to overcome any and all fertility blocks so you can finally get pregnant and have your baby.

You'll have epiphany after epiphany reading this book and will feel inspired maybe more than you have in a very long time.

That's because there is a part of you that already knows and has always known the wisdom I share here.

Don't ignore those nudges of insight and inspiration because they arise from the deep ancestral and maternal wisdom you already possess. Let those moments fuel you and propel you forward to take *action*.

As such it is important to be clear that nothing I instruct in this book is difficult. If anything, the path outlined here completely eliminates overwhelm, frustration, and wasted effort.

That being said, the principles and practices outlined in this book simply won't work until you actualize them by putting them into daily practice. I am certain you will find this process easy and enjoyable, especially in contrast to what I believe is the unrealistic and overwhelming advice you have likely already encountered.

What Makes This Book Different

Well, for starters, I refuse to waste your precious time as I try to impress you with all my fancy knowledge or terminology.

Instead, I'm going to teach you a *simple, straightforward, non-overwhelming* approach to amplifying the natural life-creating ability you already possess so you can conceive, carry, and give birth to your unique, beautiful baby.

The sheer volume of information on the internet and in books regarding fertility and reproductive endocrinology is to say the least, staggering.

We now have unprecedented access to libraries of data, knowledge, and research that - just 30 years ago - would have been the exclusive domain of university research labs and trained medical professionals.

Add to that the thousands upon thousands of blogs and books that delve into the scientific concepts of supplements, diet, and lifestyle, the so-called "alternative" paths of herbs, acupuncture, and other traditional medicines… and it's easy to see why it's so easy to end up with a sense of massive information overload.

I believe it is a good thing that we have access to so much information. We live in a world today where we take for granted that in a matter of seconds, we can literally have libraries of information in front of us that just a few centuries ago kings and emperors would have fought wars to obtain.

But - if you're like the thousands of women and couples I've worked with since I started treating fertility almost exclusively in 2005 (2000+ of whom went on to have healthy babies) - when you're having difficulty getting pregnant and you're looking for answers, the information can be as much of a curse as it is a blessing.

Depending on what you read, where you read it, who wrote it, and where they got their information, you're going to get a LOT of conflicting opinions and recommendations.

That's because much of what you read - even many of the things stated as fact by self-styled experts and gurus - isn't based on anything more than rumor, speculation, and hearsay.

Usually it goes like this - someone read it or heard it somewhere, wrote it into their book or blog, then four other people read that and wrote it into their book or blog, and it just multiplies from there.

I know this because every single week I see new patients in my clinic who repeat these myths to me as if they're fact. Later in the book I'll completely debunk these myths by telling you stories of real patients of mine whose seemingly "unlikely" success proved these myths to be false.

And, if you've been on this journey for any length of time you've already noticed that conflicts exist even amongst the scientific research. One study often contradicts the conclusions of another.

The problem is that studies are created by humans, meaning they're always biased to some degree. Just because those studies were conducted and reported by humans from big institutions with lots of letters after their names doesn't necessarily make them factual or accurate.

I want to be completely transparent with you: While I do respect and use the insights gained from scientific research in my clinic, and am immensely grateful for all these efforts, the method and process you learn in this book are 100% derived from real-world results I've achieved with thousands of patients. Some align with current research and some do not. I promise you they are effective as you will soon see.

You Will Be The "Proof"

I'm not writing this book to prove what I do works. I already know it works because, simply put, I've seen it work thousands of times.

Rather than spend tons of time explaining and justifying elaborate theories and models, what I'm going to do is simply show you how to awaken the innate power you already possess - and to do it with severe efficiency and precision.

Commit to following the simple, non-overwhelming process I teach in this book and I promise you this: Your chances of having a baby will exponentially increase as the effort and stress exponentially decrease and are all but eliminated.

You will begin to powerfully align yourself with nature and, once again, she will become your ally. And, because nature's creative spark lives inside you and already knows EXACTLY how to create your baby, by aligning with her you will harness an unfathomable amount of power that literally propels you forward with almost unstoppable force.

If that sounds like something you're ready to do, I'm certain you're going to love this book and the path it teaches.

This path is based on over a decade of experience in my clinic on the "front lines" where (as of this writing in 2019) I've helped over 2,200 people just like you - most of whom were over 35, most of whom felt their situation was near hopeless, and all of whom were desperate for real answers - to get pregnant and have babies.

And, I'm still doing it every single day where my team and I ensure we take the best care possible of those who reach out to us for help.

True Power Comes From Simplicity

It's important for you to know that what I teach you in this book is NOT complicated. Not in the least. In fact, it represents a complete 180-degree shift from just about everything else you've read, heard, or studied.

For some reason - and I honestly still don't know why this is - most people believe that for things to work they must be ornate, difficult and complicated.

This may be true when we're engineering cars, planes, and computers.

However, I promise you this: When it comes to nature creating new life inside you, the process is anything BUT complicated. It may seem so to us when viewed from an analytical, scientific perspective but, to Nature, it's not complicated at all.

That's not to say what I'm about to teach you doesn't require some focus, discipline, and a willingness to try new things and step into a different way of caring for yourself. There are certainly things you must do differently.

But I want you to rest assured that this book is not about doing 1,000 things hoping something will work.

It's about doing only the most powerful and effective things, and doing them with a fierce, but gentle, focus.

It's about committing to the simple, small changes that yield big results. It's a way to optimize and simplify. It's about getting bigger results by doing LESS, not more.

That's because what I've learned in over a decade of clinical practice is this: You don't really have to do that much if you're laser-focused on the things that truly clarify and amplify nature's power.

You Embody Unfathomable Creative Power

If you're like I once was, you've largely forgotten just how powerful and intelligent nature is and the fact that you are a literal embodiment of this power and intelligence.

You've bought into a belief that your body is like a machine and that it breaks easily and - when things go wrong - you must find exactly what to fix or it will never heal.

It's not your fault you believe that. That's what 99% of us are taught about our bodies in school. It's even what medical students are taught - that the human body is a fragile, unintelligent machine, that is prone to error and illness and rarely does things right.

Nothing could be further from the truth.

Your body is intelligent beyond anything you can imagine. It is powerful and able to overcome unimaginable obstacles even when things are far from perfect.

And I know this because I've seen it proven over 2000 times by women I've personally worked with who have conceived, carried, and birthed beautiful babies despite what seemed like insurmountable challenges.

6

And, the reason I have so much confidence in what I'm going to teach you is that pretty much all the people I've helped so far were NOT the "easy" cases. All of them had been trying for months or years to get pregnant. A large number had attempted one or more IVF cycles that didn't work. Some of them had even tried donor eggs without success.

On one level or another, they'd all been told it would be unlikely they'd have a baby, that their odds were not good, and that they had a difficult road ahead.

Yet, they all had babies anyway. They "beat the odds", so to speak.

And, the formula that got them there is as simple as it can get, laid out for you here in this book.

Follow it, and you will be amplifying nature's power in your body just like my patients did. And you'll do it using simple, concentrated, but practical steps and routines - that *anyone* can do - that represent a systematic, proven, and powerful way to strengthen nature's ability to express its life-creation blueprint through you.

That's because rather than anxiously obsessing on fixing problems, we reclaim our power and learn how to *embody the solution.*

And, this singular, relentless focus is what opens the door for nature's unfathomable intelligence to come through and do what it already knows how to do - create life inside you.

Amplifying What Is Already Perfect

When you turn your focus away from fixing what's wrong and instead towards supporting and strengthening what's right, nature always takes care of the rest.

Nature always knows how to finish the job. It has done it billions of times, over and over, and I know it can for you.

And, I will teach you exactly how to do it. I will teach you how to wake it up, clarify its path, and amplify its power inside of you.

Once nature's power has free and unfettered access to your cells, organs, and tissues, it fixes every single problem on its own, every time.

And, the beautiful thing is when you are aligning with the natural healing intelligence in your body, you don't have to do it anywhere NEAR perfect for it to work.

That's because, as you'll learn via the stories you'll hear throughout this book, nature can do *a whole lot* with "good enough".

You just have to give nature enough strength and room to operate, then get out of the way and let it do the rest for you.

I've seen this method work for countless women who were told they were likely never going to get pregnant, including:

- Sandy, who was 43, had an FSH over 80, and got pregnant after she ovulated on day 8 of her cycle.
- Julie, who gave birth to a beautiful daughter despite having had 5 miscarriages and being told she'd need a surrogate.
- Kathy, who gave birth to a son after being told her AMH was so low she needed IVF right away and there was less than a 10% chance it would work.
- Martha, who got pregnant and had a beautiful girl despite PCOS so severe she didn't even ovulate with clomid and barely had 2 periods a year.

- Jackie, who naturally conceived her son after 4 failed IVFs and 2 failed donor egg IVFs.
- Lisa, who now has a beautiful daughter she birthed at 41 and, as of this writing, is 44 years old and about to deliver her son at full term.

These, and the over 2,000 stories like them I've been privileged to witness over the last 14+ years, are not for me to show off or brag about my accomplishments. Not at all.

Each of these women simply trusted me enough to follow my guidance. They did the work. They did the simple things I taught them and let me help them a little bit.

Nature did the rest.

Their stories are here to inspire you to know that you too can overcome what seems like long odds when nature's power is strong enough and has the space to operate within you.

So, if you're ready to learn this simple way to give yourself the *best* possible chance to finally get pregnant and have your baby *regardless* of the obstacles that stand in your way, then I want to say, "Welcome. You're in the right place."

Now, let's begin.

Part One - Reclaiming Your Power

"Nature does not show herself, and therefore is apparent. She does not affirm herself, and therefore is acknowledged. She does not boast and therefore has merit. She does not strive and therefore is successful. It is exactly because she does not contend, that nobody can contend with her."

- Lao Tzu

Chapter 1 - The 21 Fertility Myths You Need to Let Go Of Today (And The Real Case Studies That Prove Them Wrong)

Most of what you've accepted as true about your fertility is simply not true.

I know this because in the last 14+ years I've helped over 2000 people just like you - who were overwhelmed with their struggle - to get pregnant despite the inaccurate stories they were told about their chances.

Just about everyone I see in clinic initially comes in with a story that they've read or heard about how the odds are stacked against them, how they have very little to no hope, or how they've likely missed the boat altogether.

And, for the vast majority (over 70%) of them, those stories ended up being false.

I'm going to tell you about real cases from my practice that defy the so-called "odds". People who came in believing all hope was lost who ended up having beautiful, healthy babies.

Can I promise you'll get the same results? Of course not. Your results are dependent entirely on you and your unique situation and ability along with your commitment to put this system into practice.

However, what I can say with ABSOLUTE CERTAINTY is that these are just a few of over 2,000 true stories of my patients that I saw with my own two eyes.

And, I absolutely promise you that the profoundly simple principles and practices I share with you later in this book are the cornerstone of why every single one of them (and thousands of others I've worked with) were able to do what they did - have babies despite their challenges.

Why do I feel it is important to do this first? One reason is, obviously, I want to demonstrate to you that this stuff works.

But, there's another purpose - one that is far more important.

I want you to let go of limiting beliefs about what you think is possible.

You might be asking, "Yeah but you told me earlier that my getting pregnant has nothing to do with knowledge - that it happens automatically as a result of nature doing what it already knows how to do. So, why does it even matter what I believe?"

True enough. You got me there. I'll readily admit there are many who - despite swearing on their lives they can't do it - end up pregnant. There are many who believe a lot of the myths I'm about to tell you and they STILL end up conceiving a healthy baby.

If anything, that just proves how powerful nature is. It proves that, indeed, knowledge and belief are not the final arbiters of what nature decides to do.

I want to ask you this question: Why continue to believe something that isn't true? Why continue to create resistance for yourself when you don't have to?

I've seen people spend months, even years, beating themselves up with all kinds of scary stories about their situation - only to find that these stories weren't true after all.

Stories like:

- I'll never be able to carry a baby to term.
- I'm too old to get pregnant.
- I never ovulate at "the right time" so my eggs must always be bad.
- I'll never be happy in life if I don't have a baby.
- My husband will be so disappointed and maybe even leave me if I'm not able to have a baby for us.
- And on and on...

Here's the thing with these stories - until it's game over, you have no idea whether these are true for you or not.

What I can tell you is I know for sure that all the above stories, along with the others I'm going to tell you below, ended up being false for over 2000 of my patients.

It's time to erase these myths from your storybook.

Oh - and one more thing...

I'm not going to get into the precise details of every single case as far as exactly what we did.

I want you to focus on the stories first because later we'll be getting into the core principles and practices they ALL followed. The entire path, every single step, will be revealed.

Myth #1 - It takes a long time - like three months or twelve months - to improve your egg quality.

There's probably no bigger misconception in the fertility world today. I can't tell you how many people I see who have read or heard this and assume it's true.

This especially comes up when I see IVF patients because they'll often come to me a month or less before they're going to start a fresh cycle. They'll say - "I read it takes three months to really make a difference with my egg quality. So, is it too late?"

The answer is a very emphatic no. Here's how I know this.

In 2008, Mindy - a 36-year-old with no children and unexplained infertility - came to me 1 week before her 3rd fresh IVF cycle. Neither of her first two cycles - the last of which was the previous month - produced a blastocyst. She was told she had poor egg quality and they would try one more time with her own eggs before moving to donor.

On the next cycle, Mindy ended up having 3 blastocysts and she got pregnant. She now has two boys - one from that cycle and one from a frozen transfer from the same batch of embryos.

Then there was Sandra. She'd been told from the beginning she'd need donor eggs. She was 39 with a very low AMH. She tried IVF on her own the month before with no eggs retrieved at all. She asked her doctor what else she could do. Because her doctor knew about me, he told her to come see me.

We started working together about 3 weeks before her next IVF procedure. She got two blastocysts. After a fresh transfer, she found out she was pregnant and later delivered twins.

14

So, what happened here? How is it that, in such a short time (weeks not months), these women were able to have such a dramatic turnaround in their results?

It's actually very simple.

There's a LOT that goes on with your eggs in the last 20 days of maturation. In fact, the follicle - which is the fluid capsule around the egg - increases in size more than 30x during the last 20 days of the maturation process. That's due to a massive influx of fluid into the follicle during those 20 days.

And that fluid contains vital hormones and nutrients that feeds and nourishes and protects the egg.

That fluid can also contain things that harm the egg or impede its normal development. Toxins, inflammatory chemicals, too much or too little of a certain hormone… there are tons of ways the follicular fluid can be out of balance and cause problems.

But, remember, with what I'm going to teach you later, we recruit nature to handle that for us. So, I don't want you to get worried about it at all.

We will harness nature's intelligence to rebalance the follicular fluid, so it conveys nature's intent with maximum efficacy.

On top of this, in the moments just before it is released by the ovary (what we call ovulation) your egg undergoes its final stage of meiosis - meaning the chromosomes separate and prepare for fertilization.

Think that's a critical time?

It certainly is. In fact, in that process that takes just a few hours the eggs chromosomes can become damaged or misaligned merely because the environment in which the chromosomes are separating isn't clear enough.

What I've seen over and over is that we can have a profoundly positive impact on egg quality in two weeks or less just by doing simple things to boost the quality of the body fluid and specifically the follicular fluid.

And remember - again - nature knows how to do this. The Clear Path is all about massive amplification of nature's power.

So, don't worry. Nature's already got it all figured out. All you must do is give it a little help.

Myth #2 - AMH is a fertility test.

Here's what we know about AMH: It is secreted by primordial follicles in the ovaries. These are the tiny little follicles that are in their most early stage of development.

I don't want to get too far off track here but, just in case you didn't already know this, you were born with about 500,000 primordial follicles, (give or take a few hundred thousand or so).

The current prevailing scientific theory is that the more antral follicles you have, the higher your AMH. The fewer antral follicles you have, the lower your AMH.

Therefore, it is thought that low AMH correlates to low ovarian reserve - meaning that there aren't a lot of follicles left.

But, here's the thing - it's NOT a fertility test. It's NOT a test of egg quality.

True, many of the people who show up in fertility clinics have low AMH because they're either over 35 and are naturally starting to run a little low on follicles OR they are under 35 and may have started off with fewer follicles than average for their age.

But I can tell you beyond any shadow of a doubt that low AMH does not equal low fertility.

Take the story of Jenny - one I've seen play out many, many times over the last decade plus.

A 39-year-old high-tech engineer, Jenny came to me after trying to conceive for almost two years. She already had a son that was almost 4 years old at the time. Initially, she wasn't in a hurry because she conceived easily at the age of 35 and figured things would be fine.

After the first year of trying to get pregnant, yet not conceiving, Jenny thought because of her age, getting pregnant this time around was going to take a little longer. She was concerned but not freaked out.

After the second year of not conceiving, she started to worry quite a bit and went to see her OB/GYN who ran an AMH test.

It came back at less than 0.16 - which for all purposes is "undetectable". Her antral follicle count (the count of follicles seen on ultrasound at the beginning of her cycle) was also low.

She was shocked as the OB/GYN told her it looked bleak and she should consult a specialist right away because she'd probably need IVF.

Jenny decided to come see me first. She'd heard about me through a friend. 3 months later, after getting on my program, she was pregnant. 9 months later she delivered a healthy baby girl at full term.

Why wasn't she getting pregnant before? I have no idea, to be honest.

But I suspect based on what happened that her body was very, very close to conceiving - but her eggs were receiving just enough damage to be unviable.

However, with the simple things we did (and that I'm going to teach you later), her body was able to make the extra little push it needed and a healthy egg, full of life, emerged.

So, while her AMH supposedly painted a bleak picture, the reality was anything but.

Myth #3 - You must make all these big, overwhelming changes to have a positive impact on egg quality and fertility.

I love this one because it gets into the concept of optimization, which is an idea near and dear to my heart.

Optimization means making small changes and getting big results. I learned about optimization when I was a software engineer between 1995 and 2008.

At the company I worked for, we would write these insanely huge programs - literally millions of lines of code - to run complex server networks.

Some of these programs we created would run thousands of operations on hundreds of computers in a matter of minutes. Something that would take days and days for a human being to manually accomplish.

At the end of our development cycle, we'd do what we called an "Optimization Run" - meaning we'd all go through our code and find areas that were bottlenecks. A bottleneck is where things get blocked or slowed down. It's usually one little routine or just a few lines of code.

Here's the cool thing - and this is what always amazed me. I could go through and find 3 or 4 areas that needed small tweaks. A line of code here, a few lines there… and just making those small little changes the program would literally run up to 1000x faster.

Yes, that's one-thousand times faster. Meaning something that took 10 seconds to complete before now took 1/10th of a second or less.

And - as I said before - this was after changing just a few lines of code out of millions of lines.

Sarah, a 40-year old pediatrician, came to me after three - yes THREE - failed frozen embryo transfers. Nobody could figure out why she wasn't able to get pregnant.

These were donor-egg embryos, first of all. Secondly, they had been unable to find anything wrong on any of the testing the doctors had done.

What I was able to discover about Sarah was that she had significant bowel issues that nobody had paid attention to. She was lucky if she had two bowel movements a week.

I know it sounds too good to be true, but all I did was help Sarah fix the bowel issues and she got pregnant on her next cycle and delivered a healthy baby girl at 39 weeks.

There is a reason why this worked. And, it's actually very, very simple - I'm surprised it's not more commonly known.

We'll get into those details later, in Part 3 of the book.

But, for now the point is that none of the things I recommend are Earth-shattering. None of them are rocket science. Yet, together, they form an almost impenetrable fortress of positive support for nature's blueprint to work flawlessly.

That's exactly what happened for Sarah. She changed a few things and got a big, big result - a baby.

Myth #4 - You must have a regular cycle with ovulation around cycle day 14.

This is one I love to debunk.

The textbook cycle is 28 days.

It's a "textbook" cycle because it's the number that was written into medical textbooks. And, that's the ONLY reason.

True, the lunar cycle is 28 days and, true, many, many women end up with their cycles synced up to that.

But a very large number of women aren't - and never will be - synced to the lunar cycle. They'll never have a regular 28-day cycle.

Yet, that says nothing about their ability to conceive a healthy baby.

Two of my patients come to mind.

One was Debbie. She'd been diagnosed with PCOS. 38 years old, she was - at most - very slightly overweight. Her cycles were between 38 and 45 days long.

The entire time she was working with me (which was about 5 months), her cycle was never less than 38 days and she never ovulated earlier than cycle day 24.

Yet, on the 4th menstrual cycle after starting with me, after ovulating on cycle day 28, she conceived her son.

Another is Susan. She came to me after 6 months of not having a period at all. She had what is commonly called "thin PCOS" meaning that she was in no way shape or form obese. Yet, she was lucky to have two periods a year.

We worked together for 6 months. During that time her persistent cystic acne (a common symptom for women with PCOS) virtually disappeared. Her lagging energy levels picked up considerably. And, her facial flushing went away completely.

But she never had a period.

She decided to take a break, which I agreed with. About two months later I got an email from her. She'd noticed some increased cervical mucus and decided to take an ovulation test and, sure enough, it came up positive. She wanted to let me know.

Then, about 2 weeks later I received another surprise. She got a positive pregnancy test. She now has a healthy baby boy.

Technically, Susan ovulated on cycle day 240 or so (8 months x 30 days).

And, she conceived a healthy, beautiful baby.

So much for that egg being "overcooked" as so many bloggers and other "experts" would have you believe.

Myth #5 - You must follow a "fertility diet" or some other strict diet.

It certainly helps to eat healthy but, as you have probably witnessed firsthand, for some reason there's always that person who drinks two Red Bulls a day and eats like total crap yet still gets pregnant.

What this proves to me isn't that those people are just "lucky" or somehow "breaking the rules".

To me it's just a reminder that nature is so, so strong. Our bodies are so incredibly resilient and can express nature's blueprint even when they're exposed to so-called "bad" habits and "unhealthy" foods.

I don't recommend you start drinking two Red Bulls a day or staying up until 2am every night.

However, you don't have to be anywhere near perfect with the simple diet changes you'll learn later, in the chapter about my "Sun Cycle Diet".

Marie, a 34-year-old stay at home mom, was having trouble with her second IVF - necessary due to a severe issue on her husband's side.

She'd come to me three years prior for help and had successfully conceived her son with IVF after a failed cycle.

She was - of course - 3 years younger back then. But there was no way that was the only explanation for why, on this most recent IVF attempt, she only produced 3 eggs.

Marie's diet was never that great to begin with. Even during the first IVF I was only able to get her to make modest changes. Yet, she still made it.

She confessed during our initial meeting about her second IVF that since having her son she'd been a lot more tired, so she was drinking 3 to 4 regular Cokes daily.

That was the only thing I asked her to change - to stop drinking the Cokes.

The next cycle she produced 17 eggs (vs. 3 eggs on prior cycle) and ended up pregnant with a healthy 5-day blastocyst that became her second son.

Pretty simple, right? And things were never "organic" or "perfect" by any stretch.

Myth #6 - The more supplements, the better.

Supplements can be helpful - don't get me wrong. I routinely use them in clinic, and I've seen so many cases where they have been.

But I've also seen cases where they've been a hindrance.

Supplements are powerful and they're extremely safe when used properly. But that doesn't mean they can't mess things up with your egg quality, lining, and other subtle factors that influence fertility.

Amy and I first met when she was 33 years old. She was a stressed-out project manager at an engineering firm who'd been trying to conceive for 3 years.

Amy was brilliant. Being trained as an engineer, she was all about the numbers, the spreadsheets, the research. And, she'd done her research.

She was taking quite a large number of supplements by the time she got to me. And, trust me, she had it all figured out as to why she was taking each one, almost down to the molecule.

Right off the bat, after she and I finished our initial conversation about her symptoms and history, I realized there were about 3 out of the 7 or so supplements she was taking that were probably unnecessary for her.

It took a little work on my part to convince her to stop taking them for a few months - after all she'd researched them extensively... But she agreed after I explained my rationale.

Along the way she noticed unexpected improvements in her sleep and her bowel function. This indicated, in my opinion, that the supplement regimen she was taking was causing subtle sleep and bowel issues - resulting in an ever so slight shift in her liver-adrenal axis - that was blocking conception.

Two months later, Amy was pregnant naturally.

So, in Amy's case, less was more.

Myth #7 - Your body is working against you.

This is one I hear a lot, and it's something you may have found yourself thinking.

"Why won't my body just do what it is supposed to?!"

Or, another flavor of that which is, "My ovaries hate me…" or "My uterus hates me…"

Nothing could be further from the truth.

Here's what your body does - it continually works to support what it thinks you are asking it to do.

Want to stay up late working on the computer every night until well past 10pm? Your body's going to faithfully attempt to adapt to that and work as hard as it can to give you the resources to do it.

Want to drink only sweet tea instead of water? Your body will do everything in its power to make that work, too.

Want to eat a diet full of processed foods? Your body is going to keep you alive as long as it can, anyway. That's how much your body loves you.

The key is that none of the above examples necessarily block fertility. Sometimes - in fact I'd say a LOT of the time - women conceive despite their bodies having to work twice as hard.

But the important thing here is to realize that your body is unique and just because someone else isn't having problems staying up late or eating a poor diet, doesn't mean you won't.

And, despite what you might think to the contrary, your body is ALWAYS trying to adapt, it ALWAYS wants to support you, it ALWAYS wants to do what you are asking of it.

Jamie was on the verge of giving up by the time we had our first visit. She was just removed from her 5th IVF (two donor egg cycles and three with her own eggs) and was at a point where she just felt like "my body just doesn't want to do this".

I remember thinking to myself, "Maybe she's right." After all, she went through 5 IVF cycles and still wasn't pregnant.

But she was adamant she wanted to keep trying and wasn't ready to give up. Her fertility doctor, who was a friend of mine, had told her to come see me because he had nothing left to offer.

"You're my last hope," she said.

I wish I could say that kind of pressure freaked me out. But, honestly, I relish it. Which is I guess why I ended up doing what I do.

As it turned out, 5 months later Jamie was pregnant. We're Facebook friends now and I recently saw a picture of her son who graduated kindergarten a few months ago.

Guess Jamie was wrong about her body not wanting to do it.

Myth #8 - Your fertility is "gone" or "lost."

This is a story I tell a lot because, admittedly, it's extraordinary. It's not something I see every day - or every year for that matter. But it proves a valuable point.

Diana, a 43-year-old finance executive, had just married about 6 months before I met her. She was working with a local fertility doctor doing IUI (Intrauterine Insemination) to try and conceive.

It was not an ideal situation, to say the least. First off, she was very obese and a Type II diabetic. Secondly, her FSH had been around 87 when it was checked about a week before we met. Third, she'd had irregular cycles for most of the past two or three years.

I admired her determination. She really believed she could do it.

Her doctor was pessimistic to say the least. Her FSH was way over 20 when they first met, and with her irregular cycles and diabetes, he was telling her there was all but zero chance she'd get pregnant without donor-egg IVF.

However, she insisted on moving forward to try with her own eggs. To his credit (in my opinion) he agreed to do his part, and the plan was for her to do injections with IUI.

They'd tried two times with no success, after which she got her 80+ FSH reading. She researched online and found the website for my clinic where I had a couple of testimonials from "high FSH" patients (these were FSH in the high teens at most) who'd gotten pregnant.

She came to me and explained the situation. I put her on the same diet that's in this book and gave her the same three core practices (what I now call "The Three Foundations") I describe in a later chapter.

Her next period came about two weeks later, and her FSH was down to 8. There was only one problem - she already had a 14mm follicle and it was only cycle day 3.

She took the injections, and within three or four days the follicle was 20mm and the doctor told her to take a trigger shot.

And… you guessed it… two weeks after the IUI - which was performed on the 8th day of her cycle - she found out she was pregnant.

I later met her beautiful baby girl.

So, where did Diana's fertility go? Was it gone, as the doctor suggested?

Apparently not.

Myth #9 - You must know exactly what the problem is in order to fix it.

I want to use Diana's story for this one, too.

You'll notice that I didn't mention any diagnosis in Diana's case other than her high FSH number…

Nobody had a clear explanation for what the cause of Diana's fertility issues was - except assuming she was too old and playing the "age" card.

Yes, she was 43. Yes, she was obese. Yes, she had a stressful job. No, she didn't have a regular cycle and, yes, she did an IUI on day 8 of her cycle.

And, she still got pregnant even though nobody knew - and I still have no clue - what the heck was going on.

Diana was one of those cases where I really didn't know exactly where to start so I just gave her the fundamentals of my program to start. Then I was going to see where we needed to go from there.

I figured that, just like with most of my other patients, we'd have a few months to see how things progressed then we could adjust.

What I learned in her case is that when life is ready, life just does it. I didn't have to even know all the details, and she didn't either. She just followed the program and she got pregnant.

And, to this day I don't even pretend to take ANY credit for it. I mean, sure, I gave her some basic recommendations and to her credit she was serious about implementing them.

It was her body, mind, and spirit that already knew what was wrong, knew exactly how to fix it, and made it happen.

To me, it always comes down to that in the end.

Myth #10 - There's something everyone else has that you don't.

There's a tendency to think that people we look up to are somehow "special", like they have a special gift that we could never have.

We think that the wealthiest people are somehow different than us. We think that people who are more successful than we are in their careers have something we don't. We think that people who are more fit and in shape than we are have a special skill we can't develop.

And, a lot of women struggling to get pregnant think they are missing something as they watch everyone else conceive seemingly with no problem.

Karen, a 36-year-old teacher, once lamented to me that it seemed like she was missing something. "I'm not sure what it is, but it seems like everyone else has it and I don't."

She'd watched as four of her coworkers all got pregnant - one of them TWICE - in the past 3 years. For Karen, this was a big blow to her self-esteem.

Her visits to the doctor hadn't been too fruitful for her. She wasn't getting answers and, honestly, I don't think there were answers. At least, not from any of her tests. They all came back clear.

When I first saw Karen I was puzzled, too. There were no glaring issues that I could pinpoint, although one thing I observed was that she was way overcommitted.

Not only did she teach flute in school, she taught private lessons after school 3 days a week.

I put her on The Three Foundations, and I also went ahead and used The Perfect Supplement Blueprint (which you'll learn about later) to find her areas of weakness so I could prescribe a couple of key supplements.

She found it difficult to practice the 30-Minute Growth Hormone Accelerator consistently, due to her time constraints with her after-school teaching. So, I told her maybe she should consider cutting back on that. She agreed after thinking about it because she realized she really didn't need the money. She also felt only one out of the six students she was teaching was really dedicated to the extra time.

The very next month after she cut back on her after-school, she was pregnant.

30

Apparently maybe the other teachers DID have something she didn't - which was time.

And, apparently Karen wasn't missing anything in the fertility department.

Myth #11 - Maybe it's just not meant to be.

I don't believe in fate, I believe in destiny.

Fate is something you have no say in. It's just "where you're supposed to end up".

Destiny is something you create and unfold. It is the alignment of your Spirit with your true purpose.

Reaching your destiny is optional and involves conscious choice.

To me, saying "it's just not meant to be," is a substitute for admitting part of you sees no way out and wants to give up.

It's OK to give up. It's OK to let it go. It's OK to move on.

For any reason and at any time you have the right to walk away.

But I hope it's not because you talk yourself out of success or you were afraid to fail. I hope it's simply because it's what you want to do.

When I feel it's time to move on from something, I like to say, "I'm choosing to let it go" instead of "it's not meant to be". That keeps me in my power.

31

Ashley thought her baby wasn't meant to be. She'd convinced herself that her life was meant to be child-free, and that she was only going to do this last attempt at getting pregnant - working with me - because her husband didn't agree with her and wanted to keep trying.

I remember her saying to me something like, "I already know it's not going to happen. I've made peace with it. But I'm going to do this because I know you can help me with my stress and if my husband sees me doing it at least he'll feel better."

Now, you might be wondering why I didn't just say, "Well, you should just tell your husband you want to stop and leave it at that."

I didn't tell her that because I am not in the business of deciding for people whether I can or cannot help them. I do wellness. Wellness is about people bringing out the best in themselves and if I see a sincere desire for change in someone who wants to work with me, then I'm in. No questions asked.

Ashley had a lot of stress and wanted help with it.

But there's another side of the story.

What she didn't know is that I didn't believe her for a second. I knew that deep down she was still longing for a child. I knew that she was telling herself it wasn't meant to be to comfort herself.

And, I'm not saying she was wrong for doing that. It's tough out here and we need to do what we need to do. Sometimes we need to lie to ourselves to get us through difficult times and I'm not going to begrudge anyone for doing that.

The thing is I have seen so many "hopeless" cases turn out to be anything but hopeless. So, I never listen to my patients' sad stories

32

anymore other than to let them know I understand them, and I hear them.

I totally believed Ashley still had it and just hadn't found it yet.

Sure enough Ashley eventually conceived. Not while we were working together - although she did feel our time was very productive in terms of helping her "get back to herself" as she called it.

Her email to me was ecstatic. She was beside herself and couldn't believe it and was very, very happy to be pregnant. She even mentioned that maybe it was all the work on her stress.

Who knows? I certainly believe that "getting back to herself" meant that she felt present in her body again and, in my opinion, that always helps fertility.

Myth #12 - If IVF didn't work you have no hope.

Angie was a sweet 32-year-old software project manager. She came to me while doing IVF, having been referred by her doctor.

Her first cycle had gone very poorly. Only 2 eggs and neither fertilized. If you know anything about IVF you know that for a 32-year-old woman, this is not an expected result.

She came to me to help with the next cycle. Results were a little better - a couple more eggs and two embryos - but she still did not get pregnant.

She tried one more cycle and got pretty much the same result again - two embryos, no pregnancy.

At that point, she decided to take a break.

About two weeks later she called me on the phone. Her doctor had told her she had the eggs of a 40-year-old woman, that it was very unlikely she would ever conceive, and recommended donor eggs. She wanted to know what I thought.

I didn't really comment on the doctor's opinion. I mean, what am I going to do - tell her the doctor's wrong when I've never seen her eggs in the laboratory, and he did?

I just asked her if she was ready to give up. And her answer was essentially, "No, I'm not. Not yet."

I also told her I personally have no issues with donor eggs or donor sperm, and I believe it is each couple's right to make that decision for themselves. My job is simply to help them make the most of whatever they decide is right for them. I wanted it to be clear that I wasn't recommending she NOT use donor eggs.

She thanked me for the call and let me know she still wanted to take a break and she'd be in touch once she felt ready to move forward again.

It was about a year later when I saw her again. She still hadn't conceived. By this time, I had started using what I know call "The Three Foundations," and I also had perfected my "Sun Cycle Diet." So, I went ahead and started her on these. She also took a couple of herbal supplements (this book won't get into herbs, but if you're interested, I recommend you sign up for "Clear Path Direct" OR consult a local acupuncturist).

Long story short, soon after coming back to work with me again, she fell pregnant. She has since had two children and I have met them both and they are quite the pair.

34

Point here is that she was essentially told she could not conceive even with IVF. And, she ended up conceiving both of her children naturally.

Myth #13 - Exercise is bad for your fertility.

True, excessive exercise can wreak havoc on your hormones, and in some cases, lead to infertility. But, in my opinion, this is the exception, not the rule.

We'll get into exercise later when I discuss my "Ultimate Egg Quality Exercise Plan". For now, let's just say this…

Your body was designed by nature to MOVE. And, in today's world, there's more than an 80% chance you're not moving it enough.

Most of the people I see, and probably most of the people reading this book, don't move their bodies enough.

Take Julie, for example. 43 years old (that's right forty-three) and after two clomid cycles, she still wasn't pregnant.

She came to me for help and, like always, I did my best to help her.

We got her on The Sun Cycle Diet which you'll learn about later, and she lost about 12 pounds in the first 3 months.

She was feeling great, but she still wasn't pregnant. So, after a couple more months, she decided to "move on."

At that time, I was running a lot after work. I'd go to the local park where we have a 3-mile running trail and do a lap after I finished clinic.

I remember running into Julie a couple of times there. She'd decided she wanted to get into shape. So, she and her husband were on a running routine where she was running three miles 4 days a week.

A few months later, just before her 44th birthday, Julie conceived her son.

Conventional wisdom - and even a lot of my colleagues - would have said that running would only hurt her chances, especially considering her age. PLUS, I live in Houston and it was summer. It is insanely hot and humid here at that time of the year. I can only imagine how much Julie was sweating. Excessive sweating is another mythical "no-no" for those trying to conceive.

Again, I'm going to get into more details about exercise in a later chapter, so don't think that YOU need to go run 3 miles for 4 days a week to get pregnant. I just wanted to illustrate that - in Julie's case at least - more exercise was more fertility, even at almost 44 years old.

Myth #14 - Tracking your cycle will help you get pregnant.

I am not a big advocate of charting and data collection. As you'll see later - in The 7 Sacred Promises - I'm a big believer in trust over tracking.

Sure, it's important to know when you're ovulating if you aren't having intercourse on a regular basis. And, it's not a bad idea to get a basic idea of how long your cycles are.

But I can't tell you how many people I've seen who obsessively track their cycle to the point of creating incredible amounts of anxiety for themselves. Every morning they wake up to take their temperature.

They're tracking every little thing they're eating and doing -- from the supplements they're taking, to their mood, what time they went to the bathroom… you get the picture.

And, by the time I see them they've been tracking for 10, sometimes 12 months. And, they're getting nowhere.

Tracking is about collecting data. You use the data to analyze trends and see if there's something you can change based on those trends.

Yet, if you're finding yourself nervous about every data point - like what's your temp going to be today - then, in my opinion, it's not worth it.

Martha had been tracking her temps for over a year by the time I first met her. She was eager to pull out her charts and show them to me in the binder she kept them in.

They were immaculate. I'd never seen so much data before, kept so perfectly, on fertility cycles.

The first thing that became apparent to me was that her charts were almost textbook. I had almost nothing to say about them. There was a slight delay in her temp rise after ovulation but other than that, I couldn't find a single flaw.

I suggested she stop tracking as part of our work together. It immediately provoked anxiety in her. I could tell she wasn't comfortable at all with my suggestion.

"Are you sure? I mean, I thought you would want me to keep tracking so we could figure out what's wrong," she said.

I understood how she felt because she'd worked so hard on the charts and here, I was basically telling her they were of no use going forward.

For a second, I thought she was going to walk out the door right on the spot.

I told her, "Look, you've kept such great records and those records show us that you have a pretty balanced cycle. You've done your part, now let me do mine."

She heard me after that. And, she agreed to stop tracking.

Ultimately, she didn't conceive until she finally decided to do an IVF cycle. And, when she did her IVF, she might as well have been the most fertile woman on Earth. I can't remember her exact numbers right now, but I know that she got pregnant the first cycle and she had several highest-grade embryos frozen for later transfers.

What's my point? My point is that all that immaculate tracking didn't solve her problem at all. Because her problem wasn't her fertility to begin with.

Does it mean nobody should ever track anything, ever? Of course not.

Just don't confuse tracking with taking necessary action to move forward on your journey. It can feel like just by tracking you're doing something. But, if you're just collecting data for the sake of collecting data, that, in many cases, is meaningless.

There's another reason I don't recommend charting cycles anymore.

Because I've seen repeatedly how people with the most imperfect cycles end up producing the most perfect babies.

Myth #15 - You need to lose a bunch of weight to get pregnant.

There's no doubt that, if you're significantly overweight, losing weight will do nothing but help increase your odds of conceiving.

It's been demonstrated in study after study that pregnancy rates are lower in women who are obese - whether that's women trying on their own or women who are doing IVF.

The reason for that is simple. The hormonal environment in an obese body is overstressed by many different factors, often shifted towards excessive estrogen (which can have negative impacts on ovulation and thyroid function).

The eggs and uterine lining often won't mature properly in this kind of environment.

But, if you are overweight, you may not have to lose much weight to get to that place where you can get pregnant.

Teresa's case illustrates this point beautifully. She'd been through 3 fresh IVF cycles when I first met her. All of them had failed. At 38 years old she was starting to worry that maybe she'd never have a child.

Teresa was very obese. She'd had a lot of trouble losing weight, too. While she wasn't diabetic, she did have mild insulin resistance. People with insulin resistance have a harder time losing weight because their metabolic system is literally slowed down on every level (again, more on that later).

So, I put Teresa on my Sun Cycle Diet and Three Foundations. I also did get her on some key supplements to balance her metabolic system (we'll get into the supplements in a later chapter).

Over a period of about two months Teresa lost 15 lbs, which for someone her size was essentially nothing... Teresa weighed around 240 lbs before, so that was less than 10% of her body weight.

Yet, on her next IVF, she broke through and got pregnant.

I've seen many other overweight patients of mine who'd struggled to conceive both naturally and with IVF end up getting pregnant and having babies after losing a relatively small amount of weight.

Your body knows your "fertile weight," or its ideal weight for conception, so don't assume you need to be "The Biggest Loser" to get there.

Myth #16 - There's an infertility epidemic caused by toxins in the environment.

Here's the bottom line (and some people are not going to like what I'm about to say):

This is not an infertility epidemic.

There is an epidemic of people waiting to have children a lot longer than nature intended.

It's only been within the last 50 years or so that it became socially acceptable for women to insist on birth control - either by saying "no" or by taking the birth control pill.

This gave women a lot more power than they had previously in terms of deciding when to start their family.

But with that power came an unintended consequence - which was that nobody wanted to talk about the fact that in many cases even waiting until your early 30's might cause trouble.

Nature brings a girl's first period when she's about 13 years old, give or take. Within a few years, she's in the prime of her fertile life.

Biologically speaking, this is a very smart thing because even just 100 years ago, average life expectancy was just a shade over 35 years.

And, as recently as 1950 we were "above average" if we lived past 48.

In other words, until recently if you wanted a decent shot at being a grandparent, you'd better start having kids when you were very young.

So, the prime biological age to have children is about 16 years old to the mid-20s.

This isn't an epidemic. It's a choice.

Another thing that's different about today is that in our industrialized society we no longer need a big family to survive. Back when most of us lived outside cities, in remote areas as hunter-gatherers and farmers (which was just a few minutes ago in Earth time), we needed large nuclear families to help with the daily work of survival like growing crops, hunting for food, and caring for both the young and the old.

41

Today, we can afford to wait to have kids because - well - we really don't need them anymore. They're a luxury. We can drive to the grocery store and get food. We can get in our cars and go to any number of places to meet with friends and socialize.

Just several hundred years ago you might live out in the middle of nowhere in a small tribal or village setting and barely see more than 20 - 30 other people for your entire life.

I've got statistics to back up what I'm saying, too (although I'm not huge on statistics because I believe they're often skewed and inaccurate). The rate of infertility amongst married couples in the United States was around 8% in the late 1800's.

Guess what it is today? Yep - 8%.

Even with all our pollution and pesticides and heavy metals the rate of couples who can't conceive is about the same.

The question is, why?

It's because nature is a lot more powerful than we think. We're so disconnected from nature we forget how much it can overcome.

I'm not saying toxins can't cause problems. For instance, it is a fact that strong ammonia and formaldehyde fumes can lead to serious problems with a pregnancy.

There's also evidence that a chemical called BPA can hinder fertility.

But I honestly think that, after over a decade of working in Houston, Texas, one of the most polluted cities on Earth due to our proximity to the largest collection of oil refineries on the planet, the toxin argument is overblown.

42

True, you can always benefit purchasing organic whenever possible (although organic won't keep you from being exposed to non-pesticide pollutants in the air and soil). And, if you want to pay a lot more for cosmetic and other products that are more natural, I am all for that.

I just haven't seen where it's made an actual difference in any of my patients' outcomes.

Later I'm going to teach you the simple, basic, powerful things you can do to enhance nature's power which, in my view, are far more effective than focusing on - and freaking out about - how toxic the world is.

Myth #17 - Plastic water bottles are making people infertile.

I'm going to be blunt on this one. It's not the water bottles that's the problem. It's dehydration or drinking things other than water that's the problem.

I know this one is going to cause some controversy, especially amongst some of my peers who strongly believe in the recent research on BPA, or Bisphenol-Alpha, as a major cause of fertility problems.

But, here's my point. Plain and simple, I don't think the levels of BPA most people are exposed to is enough to cause infertility.

I DO, however, think that dehydration can cause infertility and - as I stated earlier - I believe that the most common cause of infertility is NOT toxins in the environment, but simply poor diet and poor lifestyle habits coupled with age.

We all want to find the magic bullet - to find that one thing and say, "AHA! That's it! I've found the culprit…"

In this case, I believe it's just a way to point to something other than the obvious.

Here's the good news about this. There's a LOT you can do to overcome the things I mentioned above - namely poor diet, poor lifestyle habits and, yes, even age.

The Three Foundations, which I'll teach you later, are three of the simplest things you can ever do to strengthen your natural ability to conceive by overcoming the most common dietary and lifestyle blocks.

So, I simply don't want you to spend too much time stressing about plastic water bottles. Use common sense. If you can get all the non-plastic-contaminated water you need without causing too much stress or trouble, then by all means do so.

Otherwise, focus on what's more important which is keeping yourself well-hydrated - which will give you way more net gains than losses even if there IS a little BPA in the water.

Myth #18 - Stress makes you infertile.

You've heard it before…

- "Maybe you just need to relax…"
- "Just go out and get drunk and you'll get pregnant…"
- "My husband and I went on vacation and that's how we got pregnant…"
- "Maybe you should quit your job…"

Here's the thing - stress doesn't make you anything. It doesn't make you sick, it doesn't make you age faster, it doesn't make you infertile.

It's the way you choose to respond to stress that determines how your physiology changes.

You can go on vacation, quit your job, move to an ashram and do nothing but yoga and chant 12 hours a day… But, if you don't change how you're thinking about and reacting to life, your internal environment isn't going to change one bit.

I see this all the time. People come to me telling me they just changed jobs to reduce their stress. Within three months they're just as stressed - but about something else. Maybe at their old job it was the hours. At their new job it's a coworker that they allow to get under their skin.

One of the key practices I'll show you later is Transforming Stress Into Fertility. It's a technique that teaches you how to transform the energy of stressful states into positive energy that instantaneously shifts your body into a powerful self-healing state that supports optimal egg quality and all other reproductive systems.

Once you get to that chapter, I strongly recommend you put the technique into practice. It is, without question, one of the most powerful ways to amplify fertility I've ever encountered.

Tina was, and still is, one of my favorite patients I've ever worked with. She's a straight shooter, to say the least. She would always make me laugh with her wit and insight.

Tina doesn't pull punches, she calls it like she sees it. And, she wears her emotions on her sleeve. You can't get away with any BS with Tina. No sir.

And, that includes her husband, with whom she's had an up and down relationship.

Tina was referred to me by a fertility doctor friend of mine after a couple of failed IVFs which she was doing because of her husband's untreatable low sperm counts.

Once we started working together, she was able to get pregnant with her beautiful daughter (who I've met several times since and is adorable).

I'll never forget the day before the embryo transfer where she finally got pregnant. Tina stormed into the room. She was furious. I thought initially she was mad at me because I was running late that day.

Turns out she'd just had a big blow up argument with her husband. "F this," she said. "I'm not doing the transfer. I hate my husband and I don't want to have his baby!"

Now, I knew Tina. I knew she had a temper and there was a serious possibility she was telling the truth. But I recommended we go forward with her acupuncture session that day.

In fact, I remember after she told me her plan (and I have no idea where this came from) I just deadpanned to her, "Well, let's just do the treatment anyway, in case you change your mind."

To which she quickly replied, "Well, alright. At the very least I'll be a little more relaxed after the treatment."

So, she got up on the treatment table and I did my usual pre-transfer acupuncture protocol.

She got pregnant that cycle, as I mentioned earlier. As history would have it, even though she was still mad as hell at her husband, she went through with it anyway because she realized she really wanted a baby and she wasn't going to let this stop her.

BTW, they're still married, and they now have a son, whom I was also honored to help with when she went back for another round of IVF.

Point here is that Tina was far from "relaxed" in the traditional sense the day of that embryo transfer that finally yielded her first of two children.

She may not have been relaxed, but she certainly was REAL.

That's why I never tell my patients to "just relax". I let them feel their feelings and be authentic. I still give them the meditations and the breathing exercises, but I feel it's more important for them to be real about how they feel than to try and put a fake happy face on (which is probably more stressful than the stress itself).

Myth #19 - There's a test nobody's done on you yet that's going to detect the problem so it can be fixed.

If you've had all the tests, and nobody's yet found a reason - or even if they DID find a reason and fixed it - and you're still not pregnant… it can be insanely frustrating and demoralizing.

It's easy to start to wonder… "Do I deserve this? Have I somehow brought this on myself? Am I being punished? Am I just not meant to be a mother?"

Sometimes we never know exactly why things happen the way they do. Sometimes things just can't be explained by scientific tests.

This is where I go back to trusting nature. To sticking to what we know works, and getting back to simply supporting nature's incredible, unfathomable power.

People often go in circles for months - years even - looking for a specific reason why they can't get pregnant. Saliva tests, dried urine tests, blood tests, nutrient tests, food-allergy tests - and still no baby, no pregnancy.

Then, I go through their history and there are at least two or three obvious areas where they're just not in sync with nature's rhythms. Maybe they're going to sleep super-late or eating out of sync with the sun cycle or they're barely drinking enough water.

There's not a test for that.

Sharon came to me with all her tests in a folder. She'd had all the tests I mentioned above and more. There were a few things on them that were slightly "off" - like her adrenal cortisol saliva test showed some issues, and her food allergy test was showing a lot of stuff in the red.

She'd started on some supplements to correct the cortisol issues and was completely avoiding all the recommended high-allergy foods.

She never felt that bad to begin with, but she did say she felt a little better once she started on her new regimen.

However, after several months, she still wasn't pregnant. So, a friend told her to come see me and see if there was anything I could add.

Sharon's habits left a lot to be desired. She didn't have much of a bedtime, per se, so she just went to bed sometime between 10pm and

1230am, depending on what was on TV that night (meaning she watched TV in bed).

Her hydration was also very inconsistent. Some days she drank more, some less. Almost never did she get anywhere close to even 2 liters a day.

Another thing that nobody had picked up on (because it didn't come up on any of the tests) was that Sharon had what appeared to be some significant metabolic issues. These were "sub-clinical" obviously because the tests didn't show any pre-diabetes or insulin problems.

But when I asked her she told me that she often felt tired after meals - especially lunch.

So, without any additional tests, I recommended The Three Foundations and The Sun Cycle Diet (two of the most fundamental aspects of my program). I also put her on a key supplement to stabilize her metabolic system.

Several months later she conceived and now has a healthy baby boy.

There wasn't another test. There was no magic bullet. Nature just needed help, and once she found someone who listened to her and what her body was saying instead of running more tests, she was able to give it that help.

Simple as that.

Myth #20 - IVF is "unnatural".

Many people delay their childbearing because of unfounded fears around IVF.

Felice was one of those people.

Her husband had done a vasectomy reversal about 18 months before I first met her. She was about to turn 35 so wanted to make sure she was doing everything possible to help herself conceive as soon as possible now that her husband's sperm counts had returned to an acceptable level.

My first concern with Felice was that even though her husband's sperm counts were in the "normal" range, they were far from great. Not that I haven't seen cases where low-range normal sperm counts were enough to create a baby, but I felt his history of surgery was a red flag.

The second thing I worried about was that Felice very emphatically stated "I will NEVER do IVF. It's just not natural and I am against it."

I asked her if that was for religious reasons to which she replied that it was not. She just felt that she should conceive on her own or "I'll assume it's not meant to be, and we'll just adopt."

You'll read a little later how I feel about the whole "it's not meant to be" thing.

To me, the kind of attitude Felice - and so many others - have about IVF is based in fear of the unknown (aka "control") and fear of being judged (aka "shame").

I understand. And I would never tell someone not to follow their heart and stick to their principles.

I just think it's important not to do so out of fear and shame, but after clearly assessing the situation and gathering the facts.

And, as far as I'm concerned, IVF is not at all unnatural.

True, there's the part where the female takes medicine to stimulate her ovaries to produce more eggs. However, that medicine is a natural hormone and it stimulates a natural process of follicle growth.

Secondly, fertilizing an egg, even with ICSI (where the sperm is injected into the egg) is no less natural than planting a seed in the ground.

I don't think anyone would try to argue that it is against nature to go out in your yard, or a park, or anywhere for that matter, and plant a seed in the ground.

True, that plant may not have grown there otherwise, but how is the process not still part of nature?

I think people do themselves a HUGE disservice by taking IVF off the table before they really understand what it is.

IVF is "In-Vitro Fertilization", meaning that everything is being done by nature other than the split-second process that initiates fertilization.

Follicle growth - nature. Egg maturation - nature. Embryo development - nature. Implantation - nature. Embryo becoming fetus becoming baby becoming walking, talking human being - nature.

Here's what eventually happened with Felice. After two years of trying on her own - both naturally and with IUI (which still depends largely on her husband's sperm function) - she finally was able to hear me out on IVF.

I didn't tell her I thought she "should" do IVF. I just asked her to let me explain it to her from my perspective - someone who has seen thousands of people do it.

After hearing me out she went forward with it. It wasn't anywhere close to the disaster she imagined. She didn't go crazy from the hormones or suffer any other problems, and there were no complications.

This past year she gave birth to beautiful boy-girl twins.

Myth #21 - The solution must be complicated

I hope that by now you're already over this one.

Pretty much all the stories I mentioned above involved straightforward, simple solutions. That's because all those patients of mine followed the very simple, straightforward recommendations I gave them.

Am I claiming to be some kind of genius or magician here? Absolutely not.

If anything, I have become the anti-genius because I have stopped trying to be complicated and fancy. I've learned to trust in the simple and to rely on the power of nature embodied in every one of my patients.

I used to want to solve these big complicated problems and hence, I would come up with these big, complicated solutions.

And, it's not like these solutions never worked. They did sometimes.

But, as I progressed in my experience and understanding, I started to see that, in essence, the problem is the same for everyone.

And, if the problem is the same, the essential solution is the same.

See, the bottom line is this: Fertility is, by definition, simply an expression of surplus energy.

Your body will always prioritize YOUR survival first, and only when it knows you are OK will it devote the energy and resources to the survival and growth of a baby inside you.

Therefore a 21-year-old will conceive and birth a healthy baby even if she is severely abusing her body with drugs or other very unhealthy habits. Despite all the damage, her body has so much surplus energy (or, "regenerative capacity" as I'll refer to it later) it easily completes the conception and gestation process.

Essentially, her eggs and ovaries can withstand the abuse because they - like all the other cells and tissues inside a 21-year-old body - heal very, very fast.

That same girl 15 or even 20 years later - even if she's no longer abusing her body - will potentially (but not always) have a lot more trouble conceiving simply because she no longer has that surplus energy.

Her body simply doesn't heal as fast or as easily as it once did, and as a result more of its energy must be devoted to simple, everyday life processes.

As that surplus energy wanes, nature is no longer able to complete the blueprint it already knows, just like a person who has a precise map of how to get from point A to point B still won't get there if they are malnourished and unable to physically walk the distance.

"OK, Chris, but what about younger women with PCOS or other conditions that block fertility?"

Same thing applies, in a sense. These younger women do have ample surplus energy, it's just being used up doing things like processing the excess hormones, inflammation, and other things generated by these conditions.

In this case nature has the map and the nourishment and physical strength to complete the journey... But, for various reasons we'll easily deal with later, it just keeps veering off course somewhere between point A and point B.

The good news is that with the things you're about to learn, not only will the surplus energy be restored to the fullest possible level, your body will start to follow nature's map with a lot less effort and a lot more precision.

In other words, you'll be building massive reserves of energy and all that energy will be channeled into giving you the BEST possible chance to complete YOUR journey to having your baby.

So, what I teach here works whether you've been diagnosed with PCOS, Diminished Ovarian Reserve, Recurrent Pregnancy Loss, Endometriosis, or Unexplained Infertility.

If you have functioning ovaries and a relatively healthy uterus, this method can be a huge game-changer for you. I'm certain of it.

Of course, I can't guarantee you'll have a baby. If I could make that decision, I'd be God and we all know I'm not that.

But I will guarantee you this - follow the steps in this book and you'll be exponentially more likely to get pregnant than you are now.

And not only that... you'll be a lot calmer and happier when you arrive at your destination.

I've seen this work for over 2000 of my patients at this point.

And, I know it can work for you.

So, keep reading because you'll learn the entire process in the rest of this book. A process that has been proven repeatedly with literally over 2000 stories like the ones above.

See you in the next chapter where we'll begin breaking down the barriers and clearing the path for you to have huge breakthroughs and finally achieve your dream.

Chapter 2 - Why Nothing Has Worked Yet, And What You Really Need To Do

Here's the thing. I know how terrified you are. I know how powerless you feel. And, I know how desperately you want to find a way out.

Every time you've met an obstacle before, you've overcome it. Whether it was by using your smarts or by sheer will, you found a way.

But for some reason, this time, the smarts and strategies aren't working.

This time, it's different.

I'll tell you what's different this time. And this is key, so make sure you pay close attention.

But first I must let you know what I'm about to tell you is different from anything anyone else has told you before.

That's because not everybody wants to hear this.

And, that's for a few very basic reasons.

1. Most people only believe complicated stuff.

As I've said before, almost everyone who comes to me for help with getting pregnant, when I first meet them, believes that the solution to their problem must be ornate and abstract and massively complex or else it couldn't possibly have any validity.

Nothing could be further from the truth.

The way out of this problem is not complex, and it's not abstract. It's right under your nose and you already know exactly how to do it.

And, no, I'm not saying you're dumb for not having discovered it already. I'm reminding you of the insanely powerful intelligence you already embody, that already knows exactly how to solve this puzzle, if you just stop making it complicated and get the heck out of your own way.

And that brings me to reason number TWO that most people don't want to hear what I say…

2. Most people want someone else to fix their problem for them.

What I'm going to teach you will help you reclaim all your power, and then leverage that power to facilitate very real changes in your body that exponentially increase your fertility.

And that means you have to take full and complete responsibility for where you are, where you've been and - most importantly - where you want to end up.

Throughout this book, I'm going to tell you the unvarnished, unfiltered truth as I see it because I'm not going to play games here. You deserve better than that.

I'm calling upon you to stand up and be accountable for yourself and - by doing so - to reclaim the unfathomable power within you that is the source of all life and that knows how to create life anew.

True, there are people out here such as me who can help you… But, in the end, only YOU can change what happens inside your body.

The medicines, supplements, herbs, acupuncture, meditation, massage, and other things… these are tools to help you along the way.

They help facilitate and move things in your body. They open the door. But your cells and tissues must still have the energy and focus to be able to cross the threshold into that next chamber where conception and pregnancy are possible.

You can hire the best athletic trainer to help you prepare for the marathon. But, in the end, you're the one running it and your trainer cannot run it for you.

Which is a really awesome thing because that gives you a tremendous amount of power - especially when you have the right focus and are doing the right things.

This book gives you ALL the right things and eliminates overwhelm and confusion along the way, as has been demonstrated over 2000 times by my patients. But you must be willing to let me lead you.

So, I'm calling upon you to first allow yourself to let go of your belief this is difficult and complicated, and then to step up and take full ownership of yourself - your feelings, thoughts, choices, and actions.

And, I'm telling you to put the things I teach you into practice so you can prove to yourself they work.

Like I say to my patients all the time, "Just do this exactly as I say - for exactly 14 days - and if you aren't convinced you're on the right track, you can come tell me I'm wrong."

I've yet to have a single patient who committed to this process say they weren't feeling real, positive changes in their bodies after 14 days of doing these simple practices.

And, that brings me to the third reason most people don't want to hear what's in this book.

Again, I want you to pay attention. This is important.

3. Most people are unwilling to let go of their story about how all this is going to end up.

All that pain you're in, all that fear and hopelessness…

It's not real. It's simply the result of a scary, painful story you're telling yourself.

Initially it was a simple story. "One day, I'm going to be a mom. When the time is right, I'll stop using contraception and then I'll get pregnant."

Then, it didn't happen like that.

As the search for answers intensified, you gradually slipped into a different narrative to where now there's this constant movie playing in the back of your mind showing you how difficult, hopeless, and insurmountable this is.

And if that's what's happening, I promise, you're not alone.

- You're not alone if you're terrified inside because a part of you believes all that stuff everyone's been saying, whether "it's too late" or "maybe it's not meant to be" or "maybe you should just move on" or "just relax and forget about it and you'll get pregnant".

- You're not alone if you're telling yourself you must have done something wrong to deserve this, or that maybe you aren't meant to have a baby, or that maybe this is a sign you're not going to be a good mother.

- You're not alone if you're terrified thinking your life will have no meaning, you won't have a legacy or - worst of all - you'll die bereft and lonely if you are unable to fulfill your destiny as a mother.

- You're not alone if you've been angry, wondering why you're getting the "short end of the stick". Why is it that other people are finding it so easy yet, for you, it's a struggle?

- You're not alone if you're drowning in regret, angry with yourself, feeling like a failure because you waited until now instead of starting (or growing) your family sooner.

- And, you're not alone if you are having a hard time seeing a way out or even starting to wonder if there *is* a way out for you.

But, here's the thing. Everything I just mentioned, all those fears, frustrations, and uncertainties... *None* of them are true.

They're all just thoughts and ideas. They're all just stories you're telling yourself.

It's time to start telling a different story. Later in the book I'll explain to you why this is so important and how much power it helps you reclaim. And I'll give you a very powerful tool for doing it that has worked for so many of my patients.

See, every one of the people I worked with was like you. They were some combination of pissed off, terrified, ashamed, and overwhelmed.

They were having major doubts about themselves and their ability to get pregnant and reach their goal of starting or growing their families.

But here's the thing. My story for them was different. And my story for you is, too.

There's a story I believe to be the true story about your journey to motherhood.

And it goes something like this:

1. You are an embodiment of the most powerful creative force you can imagine.
2. That creative force *wants* to break through and do its work in your body.
3. It knows the entire process, the entire roadmap to get you from where you are now to where you want to be.
4. All it needs you to do is 3 very basic things:
    a. Strengthen it.
    b. Align with it.
    c. Get out of the way.

Something I've learned about life from observing and participating in the process of so many struggling in the realm of fertility is that - in the end - we are often our own biggest obstacle.

To that end, you'll learn some powerful daily visualizations and meditations that help you stay calm and think clearly so you don't self-sabotage or make this more difficult than it is (which is not difficult at all, actually).

Then you'll start making progress really, really fast and… the best part is… you'll KNOW you're on the right track. There will be no doubt in your mind.

More on that later.

4. Most people are looking for a "magic bullet" to avoid doing the simple (but real) work that will truly make the difference.

If you're like almost everyone I meet in my clinic, your mind is spinning with all the conflicting information you read. One book says this, the other says that. One blogger recommends this, another a completely different thing.

You read a scientific paper or a detailed report on reproductive endocrinology and by the time your head stops spinning, you don't even know where to begin.

And, even though this brings you even more anxiety, you keep doing it anyway.

Eventually searching itself becomes the problem, just compounding the sense of anxiety and overwhelm you already feel.

It's Time To Embrace Simplicity And Trust In Nature Again

Truth is there is no "magic bullet" out there. The magic bullet is right here, right now.

The "magic bullet" is YOU.

I know this with absolute certainty because I've seen it bear out over 2000 times in my clinic with women and couples who'd been told:

- They had "less than a 1% chance"
- To just "move on" or "accept God's will"
- That "maybe it's just not meant to be"
- That their egg quality was irreversibly bad
- That other problems like endometriosis, PCOS, recurrent miscarriage, thin uterine lining, early or late ovulation were going to difficult, if not impossible, to overcome.

They went into massive research mode, trying to learn everything they could about their situation, what supplements they should take, what things they should and shouldn't do, foods they should and shouldn't eat…

It's a place I call "the baby-making bunker" (which is that dark lonely room in front of the computer or smartphone endlessly researching). And, if you give them a chance, the simple practices in this book will break you out of that bunker for good.

None of what you're going to learn is fancy or ornate, yet all of it is profoundly powerful for amplifying nature's blueprint inside you.

These daily, simple routines - including dietary adjustments, supplements, exercises, and visualizations - are what has helped over 2000 of my patients transform themselves from stuck, frustrated, and terrified to calm, certain, clear, and (of course) pregnant.

You do not have to know how or why any of it works for it to work, any more than you must understand the chemical reactions happening inside the sun in order to feel warm standing in its light.

When it comes to creating life, nature's got you covered.

If you're still reading, then I'm assuming you are ready to create a new path for yourself.

You heard my story for you. The one where you embody unimaginable creative power and you learn how to awaken it, clarify it, amplify it, then sit back and watch as it gets to work taking you on your journey to motherhood and having your baby.

If you're willing to give me a chance to show you how to do it, I absolutely guarantee your life will never be the same again.

Chapter 3 - From Anxious And Overwhelmed To Powerful And Pregnant - The "Six Laws Of Seed Intelligence"

I want to remind you that you're not alone. Many, many people have walked this path before you. Many, many women have faced this same situation and overcome it, giving birth to their beautiful, perfect babies.

And, I completely believe in your power to join them.

But, to do so you're going to have to change some things. It's as simple as that. I don't want to sugar-coat or dance around the issue…

For whatever reason - a reason we will never fully know - you find yourself where you are right this second, reading this book, looking for a way out of the pain and helplessness you're feeling. It's not something you ever wished upon yourself and you probably wouldn't even wish it on your worst enemy.

It absolutely sucks, being in this place. You want answers but every time you think you've found one it seemingly slips through your fingers and you find yourself right back where you started.

It's what I call "The Circle of Pain", and it isn't happening to you because you deserve it or are dumb or not good at solving problems.

It's happening to you because your usual way of solving problems doesn't apply in this situation.

We're taught that to solve something we must do the research, do the math, get our precise plan together, then methodically apply our solution so that things work as we planned.

And, that absolutely works: In business, in academics, in manufacturing, in engineering and in financial planning.

But what we're dealing with here - in terms of you getting pregnant - is something that can't be controlled or tamed. It's the very creative force of life itself.

Nature does what it wants, when it wants. It does not bend to intervention in the way we normally think. Anytime we try to intervene to control nature she pushes back harder. We're often playing a losing game, or one with potentially dire repercussions.

That's because nature accepts no bargains. She can't be bribed or paid-off. She accepts no reasons or excuses.

If you're standing on a rock next to the ocean enjoying the beautiful view and a wave comes and sweeps you out to sea, nature doesn't have any interest whatsoever in your intentions, how much money you have or how smart you are. It doesn't leave you alone because you were appreciating its beauty.

It's just going to sweep you out to sea with the current because... well... that's what nature does. It makes big waves, and those big waves are very powerful and move things far out into the ocean.

And, that's it.

Nature simply does what nature does. Relentlessly and powerfully and beautifully and... yes... quite ruthlessly.

The question is simply are you going to fight this power or align with it? Are you going to become nature's ally? Or, are you going to keep trying to make nature do things your way?

I've found in the process of working with literally thousands of women just like you that there are certain "laws" that, when followed, rapidly bring us into alignment with nature and allow us to harness the power of nature inside our bodies and minds.

And it is this natural strength inside you that gives you the best possible chance of getting pregnant.

The simple exercises and daily practices you will learn in this book - from diet and lifestyle to mindset and medicine - are designed around these laws of nature, to help you harness them and leverage them for maximum benefit.

All you must do is… DO them.

Is what you're about to learn here difficult? Absolutely not.

Is it *different* than what you're used to? Most likely.

Will it require a little effort and a willingness to try new things? Absolutely.

I've seen many of my patients make this process more of a struggle than it has to be. Again, a lot of that comes from holding onto a story that it must be a struggle, that "hard work pays off", which doesn't apply in this case.

In fact, what you're about to learn is almost certainly EASIER than what you're doing now and when you follow my lead, you'll be doing 10 times LESS but getting 10 times MORE out of it.

And when you embrace simplicity and directness you become nature's creative partner and she becomes your fierce ally and protector - and this whole process stops feeling burdensome, scary, and overwhelming.

Remember this: Nature isn't going to be bought or bargained with. It won't bend to your will. If you *fight* her, you will almost always lose.

When you find a great mentor - no matter what business or field or area of knowledge you are interested in - you naturally start to absorb that mentor's knowledge and experience just by being around them... You watch them, you model them, you can literally take in their wisdom just from being in their presence.

If you've never had this experience, trust me, it's amazing. As a musician I remember when I would be in the presence of masters - whether at a concert, in a lesson, or just hanging out - and how much it would accelerate my trajectory to mastering my own instrument.

For the purposes of what you want to do - create life - you have ONE mentor, ONE teacher, ONE entity that knows the entire way and embodies all the wisdom you need.

Your mentor is Nature herself.

And, here's the really good news... She is already right here, inside you.

In other words...

You already embody the solution you seek.

So, the question becomes, "Then why then am I struggling so much? What is wrong with me? Why is it so easy for other people and not me?"

I don't know and I'll never be able to answer that question for you. And, you won't either.

As much as we all want this to fit into a neat little box and find the switch that's going to turn it all on, it never will fit into that box, and we'll never find the magic switch.

There isn't a box because while nature is orderly at times it's also messy as hell.

And there isn't a switch because nature is always running at full power.

This is why, despite all the tests, diagnostic labels, procedures, and other things people go through on this journey, a whole lot of them still aren't pregnant.

Doing IVF - for instance - is a powerful way to facilitate conception. In fact, I find it to be incredibly helpful for so many couples and I'm grateful it exists.

But, even with everything involved in the intricate process of IVF - the injections and stimulation, the retrieval and fertilization of the egg, the culturing and incubation of the embryo, the hormonal priming of the uterus and the transfer of the embryo...

Nature still does everything.

It is nature that responds to the injections, matures the eggs, sparks the fertilization process and sustains the initial growth of the embryo. Nature is what responds to the estrogen and builds that beautiful lining and makes it an inviting home for your baby.

When things don't go well, it's natural to want to figure out EXACTLY where they went wrong.

Was it health of the embryo? Was the lining not ready? Did the ovaries just not respond as anticipated? Was the body just unable to sustain the pregnancy? Was the sperm quality not up to par?

Sometimes we can get clear answers. Sometimes we can't.

But I'll tell you who always knows the answer.

Nature.

And by nature, I mean… YOU.

The answer to all these questions is inside you right now. The problem is you can't *think* the answer.

You must *embody* it.

And, once you learn how to embody the answer, there aren't any more questions.

When you follow these Six Laws Of Seed Intelligence, you align with the power that's already inside you… so you can begin the process of embodying and becoming the answer, forever escape "The Circle of Pain", and accelerate your path to having your baby.

They truly are the most powerful way I've discovered to walk the journey from struggle and fear to confidence and power.

Why Do I Call It "Seed Intelligence"?

Because by following these six principles you awaken that part of yourself that ALREADY KNOWS how to complete this process we call conception, pregnancy, and birth.

Just like a seed already contains all the wisdom and knowledge it needs to grow into the plant or tree it is destined to be, you embody all the wisdom and knowledge you need to get where you want.

When you connect with that deep wisdom, you begin to feel confident, calm, and powerful. And, I can tell you this for certain - when you feel powerful and confident again - EVERYTHING becomes easier.

All because you're connecting with a force that is already inside you.

A word of caution here… If you're the kind of person who thinks drinking water instead of juice or flavored drinks is difficult, or getting proper rest is a waste of time, or eating healthy foods is hard to do, or that taking some key supplements is oh-so-annoying, then for this to work you're going to have to be willing to let go of that story. You're going to have to stop making it hard on yourself because it's NOT hard to drink water, sleep, and eat healthy foods.

There's also this idea of "I can't meditate" or "I can't calm my mind." Again, if you want to keep telling yourself that story, it will make this process a lot more difficult. Meditating and calming your mind is incredibly easy if you'll just trust me and follow my methods.

Bottom line - for this to work, you must commit to it.

Also, you don't have to memorize The Six Laws, because the methods I'm going to teach are based upon them and encapsulate them very well...

If you find it useful you can come back to this chapter and re-read them when you feel you need to refresh or reboot yourself and get inspired again. I find them incredibly inspirational and they are quite universal in their application.

You may find yourself coming back to them long after you've completed your motherhood journey, to help you stay on track and get inspired about other things.

I truly believe they are that powerful.

So, let's (finally) get to the laws themselves. I'll explain each briefly, but I don't want to go into too much detail. They sort of "are what they are."

And, if you follow the steps in this book - including the meditations, exercises, dietary changes, supplement recommendations, and lifestyle modifications - you'll be aligning yourself with all these laws and, as a result, you'll tap into an incredible amount of power and wisdom you never imagined you had.

That's because you will begin to more fully embody the truth of your own power - you as a creative spark within nature.

1) The Law Of Desire

"Desire is the fuel of all change. It is the fire that propels us forward and lights the way to our destiny."

72

This is important. You must really, really let yourself want this.

"But of course I do… Of course, I really want this. How can you question my desire for a baby?"

I'm not questioning your desire. I'm simply saying you must allow your desire to be full, to be open, to be REAL.

"But people get pregnant all the time without wanting to… Why are you telling me it has something to do with desire?"

Because for YOU, it does. Otherwise you wouldn't be reading this book.

You're going to have to stop thinking about what everybody else wants or doesn't want. Or what happens in the lives or minds of others.

The only thing that counts here is what YOU want. The only thing that is going to carry you through to your destination, through every trial you face, is *your* desire.

And, you must want it with all your heart. You must let yourself feel that desire without fear.

You see, so many people - in so many ways - hold back their desire. They know they want something, but they're so afraid of the pain of not getting it that they hold back their hope and, with it, their effort.

I want you to fully open to your desire. To be able to scream with all your might, "HELL YES I WANT THIS. I WANT A BABY."

And, I want you to let go of all justifications and rationalizations for holding back your heartfelt desire to be a mother.

You see, rational and logical just don't help here. Not one bit.

Having a baby is a HEART desire, not a MIND desire. It is a desire rooted in unconditional love. Period. End of story.

When you truly let yourself WANT this, you suddenly open the floodgates of an immense amount of MOTIVATION - which is what you will need to MOVE FORWARD with the kind of force that it is going to take to get where you want to go and to make the changes necessary to align your life with nature so that it can bring new life into you.

Raw, unfiltered, pure, heartfelt desire - free of guilt or shame or fear - is the rocket fuel that will propel you on this journey faster than you can imagine.

And you must go full throttle.

Do not be afraid to fail. Be afraid of holding back. Be afraid of not allowing yourself to really, really want this.

I'm a big fan of seeds, which you'll discover as your read this book.

A seed does not question its desire to reach for the sun, to root down into Earth. It contains the entire blueprint to become the fullness of what nature intended, and it fearlessly, shamelessly, relentlessly, and (most important) effortlessly seeks to fulfill and complete that blueprint.

Be like the seed. Stop questioning who you are and what you want. Go forward with complete passion and purpose... Reach - with all your heart - for your destiny as a mother, if that is truly what you want.

I'll help you align with the Law of Desire using a simple exercise I call "Own Your Story", which is also a great way to energize and reconnect with positive, uplifting, joyful energy.

2) The Law Of Acceptance

"It is impossible to change what we refuse to embrace. Accept who you are and where you are, right here, right now."

There's nothing we can do to change the past, and there is nothing we can do to change the fact that you have arrived at this moment and have entered this struggle.

- All those babies you see everywhere.
- The friends and family members who are, were, or will be pregnant before you.
- The hurtful comments and advice you keep hearing and reading.
- The pain inside your heart and the fear, frustration, and worry that feeds it.
- The feeling of helplessness because there's no guarantee of success.
- The loss of control and feeling like your body has turned against you.

Accept it all, right now.

You're not accepting it in the sense of giving up or resigning yourself.

You're accepting it because it's time to stop fighting. It's time to stop running away.

It's time to stop wishing things were different.

Change must start right here, in this moment. And, if you can't BE in this moment it is impossible to change it. Simple as that.

By accepting yourself and your situation, you let go of the desperation and the suffocating anxiety. You are no longer hiding from your pain. And that frees up an *enormous* amount of energy.

One of the now-classic American movies, Shawshank Redemption, is a movie about the kind of acceptance I am talking about here.

Andy, the protagonist, is given a life sentence for a murder he didn't commit. At first, he is in shock and completely rejects his fate. But soon he begins to understand that if he ever wants to escape, he's going to have to settle into life where he is, learn the ropes, and patiently take the necessary steps to gain his freedom.

The turning point of the story is when he finally overcomes the desperation to escape RIGHT NOW. Once he accepts where he is, ironically, it is that moment when he can begin truly working towards his eventual escape.

Day by day, little by little, Andy literally "chips away" at the wall in his cell, devising a plan for his eventual escape. And, once he starts to realize his plan is working, he finds joy and solace even as he completes his days behind bars.

That's because he realizes that, indeed, he WILL escape. And you will realize this too once you put the steps I teach you into action. You will begin to KNOW you are on the right path. You will feel it with every cell of your body, and it will bring you immense joy and inner peace.

Your path from overwhelmed prisoner of a seemingly endless struggle to a calm, confident liberated spirit starts with our first meditation exercise later in the book, called "Inner Space / Inner Peace."

3) The Law Of Loving-Kindness

"Loving-Kindness concentrates and sustains the power of Heart, which brings peace and purpose to every thought, word, and deed as well as every cell, organ, and tissue."

Now, more than ever, you've got to show loving-kindness and mercy to yourself.

You didn't do anything to deserve this. Nor did you ask for it. You are not being punished and there is no punisher. Except for you.

The only one who is berating, judging, belittling, and shaming you is you.

I hear this all the time from my patients: "How could I have been so stupid to wait this long, I should have had my kids earlier."

Anyone who is having problems getting pregnant starts to question themselves and - when the answers elude them as they always do - they start to *blame* themselves.

And, what you'll find when you start seeking to blame is a mountain of hellfire coming down upon you.

"If only…." "Should have…". "How could I have…". "I'm such an idiot because…".

To get yourself on the right track, you're going to have to stop all that, resign your role as judge and jury, and take on the role of loving, caring mother... to YOU.

One of my patients had been through multiple miscarriages. She was so brutally hard on herself about it. She really felt either her body was "defective" or that she was being punished for a past sin.

I was able to have this conversation with her about loving-kindness. I was able to impress upon her the fact that nobody was buying that story, except for her. And that even if others had somehow repeated it or supported it, she was the one choosing to accept it and believe it.

I helped her see that she had the choice to focus on a different story. Right now.

The sooner you start directing loving-kindness towards yourself, the sooner you will stop filling yourself with the toxic, suppressive, oppressive emotions of shame and guilt (which we'll learn later have powerful hormonal and neurological impacts that can alter the signals that guide your fertile state).

Committing to self-directed loving-kindness - and rejecting shame and guilt in the process - is the single most liberating thing you can do for yourself.

Imagine you're back in the 2nd grade. I walk into your classroom to teach calculus. I'm writing all the equations on the board, I'm the best calculus teacher the world has ever known. I explain it with a clarity and precision that makes it really, really easy to understand.

What do you think is going to happen?

You're not going to understand a damn thing.

That's because you're in the SECOND GRADE. You simply aren't there yet. Cognitively speaking, it is *impossible* for your brain to comprehend calculus when you just learned and mastered basic addition and subtraction.

The same applies for your journey to where you are now. 3 years ago, 5 years ago... I could have given you the most logical, clear, and precise guidance around how your decisions were going to potentially impact your ability to conceive today.

And, it simply would not have computed. You simply weren't there in your life.

Ask yourself this question: Would you punish the child who couldn't do calculus in the 2nd grade?

Of course not.

So why are you punishing yourself now?

Sure, in many ways we all look grown up but in just as many ways all of us - and I mean ALL of us - are still children inside, still very much learning the basic geometry and calculus of life.

So, stop being so hard on yourself. In fact, stop being hard on yourself *AT ALL*.

Practicing The Law of Loving-Kindness is the ultimate salve for all of life's wounds, all of life's pain.

You ruthlessly, continually, and unashamedly love yourself, just like you would love that 2nd grader being chastised for failing calculus.

The psychological, emotional, spiritual, and BIOLOGICAL effects of this are powerful, profound... and necessary.

Don't wait another minute, another second. It's not worth even one more word of self-directed scorn or judgment.

I'll help you align with this law through a powerful and life-changing exercise I call "Awakening The Seed", later in this book.

4) The Law Of Unification

"When all our internal and external resources - including Body, Mind, and Spirit - are moving in the same direction at the same time, there is literally nothing that can stop us."

Up until now, whether you realize it or not, you've been dealing with an internal conflict.

The desire in your heart for a baby is strong and beautiful and pure. It is rooted in deep unconditional love you want to shower upon your future child.

At the same time, you're terrified of the pain of failure, so your rational mind tries to keep your desire in check. Can't tell you how many times I've heard, "I don't want to get my hopes up..."

All the emotional ups and downs, the research, the finding something that gives you hope then suddenly feeling lost again, these are signs that you are going in circles, that you are in some ways (unintentionally, of course) working against yourself.

And, if you're eating, hydration, and sleep habits are not at least minimally rhythmic and clear, you add another layer of fragmentation for your body to deal with.

The point here is that the best way for you to get on track is to start getting all your resources - Body, Mind, and Spirit - going in the same direction at the same time.

This is what I call "Unification." And, it's insanely powerful.

Now, before I go further with this topic I want to make something crystal clear. This is NOT about perfection.

There is no perfect diet, there is no perfect routine or lifestyle or exercise pattern or supplement regimen or... ANYTHING else.

And, that's a good thing because nature doesn't need perfection. Not even close.

Nature simply needs "good enough." Meaning that nature will break through, even in very trying circumstances, to create life more abundantly than you can imagine.

Think of the seed that falls in a small crack in the cement. What happens? It begins to grow. There might be cars whizzing by at 60 mph, there might be unimaginable noise and heat and even "pollution."

Yet, the seed sprouts upwards and grows and grows.

Soon the city road workers are being called out to trim back or remove the small tree that grew out of that tiny crack.

I remember the first time I visited New York City when I was in high school. I was on a bus traveling into the city from Newark airport and as we were going down the crowded expressway there was this fully-grown tree coming out the side of a huge concrete wall.

I guess because the tree didn't pose any danger to the cars driving by, the city hadn't gone to the trouble of removing it.

You would think that tree could never make it. Can you imagine when it was just a seedling sprouting up amid all that noise and activity, not to mention the tiny crack in the cement that was its only space to grow in?

That tree, standing there all alone growing out the side of a concrete embankment, still to this day is the image I conjure up to represent true strength and resilience. Alone, yet determined, the tree not only survived, it thrived in circumstances that were FAR from ideal.

The irony of trying to do all this stuff perfect is that you create the opposite. By pursuing perfection, you are unwittingly guaranteeing you will experience anxiety, struggle, and self-reproach time and time again. You may be driven to this choice subconsciously, but it's still your choice.

Wanting to do all this stuff perfectly does not help you do it better. Not at all. It only helps you do it with more tension, anxiety, and shame.

In other words, trying to be perfect is not the road to success. It is almost a certain guarantee of failure.

To unify your resources, you must let them be as they are. You must be NATURAL and EASY. Relaxed and free in spirit.

The example of the seed from earlier is the perfect example. It just reaches for the sun and roots down into Earth. It is not self-conscious in the least. It just keeps moving forward. If the wind blows upon it, it bends. It doesn't care how "straight" it looks. If it needs to grow "crooked" to get more sunlight, then it does that without hesitation.

The trees next to each other in a forest aren't comparing themselves to each other. They are too busy growing and being beautiful to care. Each is unique and it is their uniqueness which signifies their perfection.

The simple rituals of diet, exercise, lifestyle, and thought laid out in this book are carefully designed in a way to bring about this state of "Unification" by helping you do all the small, simple things that get everything aligned in a very natural, non-overwhelming way.

5) The Law Of Time and Space

"We create more time by slowing down. We create more space by being open."

Time and space - the two built-in limiting factors of life. We've only got so much of both and, when comes to both, you either have an abundance mentality or a scarcity mentality.

Unfortunately, most of the people I meet - and you may be one of them - have a scarcity mentality around time and space.

The mantra of someone on the time/space scarcity continuum goes something like this: "There's never enough time, and there's never enough space - for me."

People who live in what I call a "small world" are continually in a rush. Every little second counts. They're so busy taking care of "obligations" they are completely overwhelmed almost all the time.

Time/space scarcity leads to a dramatic loss of power. You put your power in everything else - your job, your status, your social engagements, your perceived obligations.

I call this "living life outside-in." It's where all your happiness is sought in the outer world of status, social interactions, and achievement.

And anyone who lives this way long enough inevitably finds that, one day, there's nothing left on the inside. No energy, no focus, no power. Nothing.

It's a very crappy place to be. I know because I've been there.

The opposite place, time/space abundance, is a whole different story.

In this place you realize that time is, in fact, an infinite resource. It goes on indefinitely, as does space. There is no limit to your time, there is no limit to the amount of space you can claim.

But, here I'm talking about *inner* time and *inner* space. I'm talking about your ability to slow down and to create healthy boundaries for yourself.

A great meditator (and *you* are a great meditator whether you realize it or not, but we'll get to that later) can sit in the middle of a busy intersection or subway station - with all the noise and chatter and rumbling - and maintain perfect inner peace.

She is not swept up in the rush of the rat-race. Nor does she feel crowded or crushed by the hustle and bustle.

That's because she has literally CREATED time and space within herself.

You can do it, too. And, it's a lot easier than you think.

The first step in this is to simply realize that by slowing down you are creating more time. It's completely counterintuitive, but it's true.

When you stop rushing around and you move through life without haste EVERYTHING slows down - your nervous system, your circulation, your brain waves, your heart waves… And, this slowing-down process not only dramatically enhances and amplifies the natural function of these critical body systems, it also leads to a more abundant, more gentle, more soothing sense of time.

This is a hard one for many of my patients to grasp because - after all - you've been told your "clock is ticking" and you're "running out of time."

True enough, there are biological limits we all must learn to accept. Nature, as I said before, can't be bought or bargained with.

Responding to this "time crunch" by rushing and hurrying is, however, the worst thing we can do both from an emotional and biological perspective. It only creates the reverse of what we intend by scattering and depleting the very resources we need most.

And, besides, it almost never works.

Nature is inherently slow. She takes her time. If we want a seed to grow from seedling to 300-foot redwood in 3 days, it's simply not going to happen. No matter how much we want it to or how we try to engineer it to happen, it's just not going to happen.

Instead of "hurry up and wait," however, in the way I'm teaching you here, we do something I call, "slow down and create."

That's because by slowing down you magnify and amplify your creative power beyond anything you can imagine.

As I said just now, NATURE IS SLOW. Therefore, the faster you are going and more frantic you are, the more you are out of alignment with nature.

I'm going to be teaching you very clear, easy-to-follow practices that help you stay calm and focused. These daily rituals powerfully awaken natural forces inside you. And, you can start doing those things today, right now.

We're not going to be passive at all. We're going to be taking very calm, measured action. And the result will be this: You will, without any anxiety or hurry, be allowing nature to "catch up to you". You'll no longer be "swimming ahead of the current", so to speak.

You'll be totally relaxing and letting the nature's gentle current take you where it already knows how to take you - to your most creative, powerful self. THAT is the version of you that is, by far, the most capable of reaching your dream of getting pregnant and giving birth to your baby.

The other part of this law of time and space is to recognize that the space outside of you will never increase. You'll never create more "outer" space.

Yet the space within you is infinite and you can create as much as you want.

That means space between thoughts and feelings, space between activities and obligations. Space for you to just BE.

I often wonder - when I first meet patients who are trying to get pregnant and who are, at the same time, working 60-hour weeks and going to night school and living busy social lives - "where is there space for a baby in there?"

You read the story earlier about the patient of mine who got pregnant very shortly after she reclaimed all that extra time she was spending tutoring her students after hours.

That was not a coincidence, nor was it luck.

It was because she changed her behavior - her actions - and Nature responded in kind.

See, as far as Nature is concerned talk is cheap.

Nature does not speak in words. Her language is movement and change. She does not care what we say. To her, our words are completely meaningless.

People can say they want a baby until they're blue in the face. They can tell everyone they know how much they want a baby. They can wake up every single morning thinking "baby, baby, baby."

But, if their actions don't align with what they're saying, it's highly unlikely they'll get what they say they want, no matter how many times or how forcefully they say it.

I'll never forget one of the couples I worked with who had struggled for many years to get pregnant. They were finally able to conceive within a short time of starting to work with me, but the pregnancy did not last more than a few weeks.

They were truly devastated. So much so that they decided to take a break from the entire baby thing.

About a year after I last saw them, I received an email. They'd decided to adopt, and they wanted to thank me for all the help I'd given them. It was such a sweet gesture and, honestly, I love when patients who DON'T get pregnant still understand the value of the caring and support they received working with me. Because, I know that is the only thing I truly control in all this - how much I care and how committed I am to giving the best advice and support I possibly can.

Anyway, a few months later another email pops up. As part of the adoption process they were getting the baby's room ready. They chose the room and had bought the furniture and were setting up the room when the wife suddenly felt dizzy and nauseous.

Yes, it is what you think it is. She'd missed her period and decided right then and there to take a pregnancy test to make sure she wasn't pregnant. And, it came up positive.

She emailed me because she was scared she might miscarry. I knew otherwise. I was so confident because now she was making space in her life for the baby (whereas before there was very little to none).

Her biology simply aligned with her actions, and boom.

She did go on to have a full-term pregnancy and they now have a beautiful son.

Because she got pregnant, the adoption process was put on hold. However, the last I checked with them they were back in the adoption game. They felt the need to complete that process because they'd truly set their hearts on giving a baby a beautiful home.

By following what I teach throughout this book, you're going to be creating both time for you to get back to center and space for your baby to come into being.

6) The Law Of Focus

"Your attention is your internal Sun. What you put your attention on grows. Learn to direct your attention towards what you truly want, and it will naturally blossom."

Struggling with getting pregnant can become a real test of sanity. The fears, the regrets, the guilt, the shame, the frustration - all the *emotions* can start to take a huge toll on your ability to maintain balance.

They're called *emotions* because they cause *movement*. They move us to act. However, when you're feeling all these deep, heavy, intense emotions which arise around the getting pregnant journey, you naturally start to feel overwhelmed.

How can you possibly move in all those different directions all at once?

The answer is - *you can't*.

So, instead you feel paralyzed, almost numb. There's an inherent shutting down that starts to take place. And, considering that when our emotions are out of control we're more likely to do irrational things, this paralysis is a good thing that, in a way, keeps us safe.

The key now is to start to move again, to get yourself into a flow and start moving forward. To get out of "analysis paralysis," and into clear, consistent *action* mode.

And, that is going to require focus.

When I first learned the law of focus, honestly it was a Godsend.

I had opened my acupuncture clinic in 2004 after working full-time as a software coder and going to acupuncture school in the evenings and on weekends for 4 ½ years.

I continued working my software job initially because, well, I had bills to pay and a family to feed. So, I saw patients in a nearby small office space, gradually building things up in my practice until, in 2008, I was doing well enough to quit my "day job".

There was one catch. While my acupuncture clinic was starting to get busy, it wasn't generating anywhere near the income my software job did.

But, I was ready to make the jump. I was already feeling the passion and excitement for my real career as a healer and I could no longer wait.

The first few months were a dream. I was making just enough money - along with the small savings I'd built for the transition - to pay my bills at home and pay my rent at the office. It was a very tight margin, but I was making it.

Then, two things happened. This was 2008 and if you are American you remember one thing for sure and may remember the other.

First, Hurricane Ike hit Houston. Now, hurricanes are no joke, as you probably know. But, this one was particularly devastating for Houston. I'd been through hurricanes and powerful storms before, but nothing like this.

About 70% of the city lost electricity, meaning literally millions of people had no power at home or at work. Gas stations couldn't even pump gas and grocery stores were closed for days.

At my clinic, we went from a schedule with 30 patients booked the week before the storm, to 3 patients booked the week after.

Yes, you read that right. 30 to 3.

And, to make matters worse, we simply couldn't reach most of our patients and the ones we could reach were completely in over their heads with damage to their homes, no electricity, and not even able to go to work.

Then, right in the middle of all that came the big market crash that started "The Great Recession" of 2008.

So, now not only did our patients have logistical problems, there were serious financial worries keeping any new patients from calling us.

I was terrified, to say the least. It took me about 6 weeks to get over the shock. It was like someone dropped a bomb on my head and scrambled my brain for those 6 weeks.

But, then I remembered The Law of Focus.

For those initial 6 weeks I was obsessing on how I was about to go bankrupt and my dream of being a successful healer and making a living doing what I loved was going to go down the drain along with all I'd worked so hard to achieve - my house, my savings, everything.

I was feeling so ashamed because I knew that I'd made a choice that didn't sit well with my family (to leave a successful career in software to pursue a career in "alternative medicine") and my imminent downfall was going to prove them right.

Then, something amazing happened.

One of the few patients who was still attending her regular sessions came in for a treatment. She'd just found out she was pregnant and, after her session, took a little time to give me a very sweet, heartfelt thank you and to tell me how much my support and my care had meant to her.

Honestly, there's probably no way she could have missed how much I was struggling to stay focused at the time. She knew what was going on in Houston, and she knew my clinic was suddenly very, very quiet when just weeks earlier it was buzzing with energy.

So, I'm certain she told me this not only because she meant it, but because she wanted to help me. And, to say she accomplished her mission would be a severe understatement.

Her heartfelt gratitude flipped a switch inside me. I suddenly remembered why I was doing this work, and it was like the fire was re-lit.

I found a level of desire I never thought I had. I decided I was going to make it work NO MATTER WHAT. That I was going to fulfill my purpose despite all the difficulties seemingly thrown at me out of nowhere.

And, I decided to relentlessly shift my focus to how I was going to help my patients. That was going to be my entire focus and from that I would know what to do.

Did I have moments where I was scared as hell? Yes, absolutely. But in those moments I would remind myself "What I focus on will grow…" and I didn't want the fear to keep growing. So, I would shift my focus back to "how do I help my patients, how do I help more people, how do I reach the people who need my help?"

Needless to say, it worked. I was able to make it through that "perfect storm" of a hurricane and a financial crisis and here we are today where (as of this writing) The Axelrad Clinic has 3 offices and 7 employees and we're helping over 200 people every single week.

And, there is no doubt in my mind the turning point was when I chose to shift my focus from what I couldn't control (the storm and the aftermath and the financial crisis) to what I COULD control (my commitment to making a difference in my patients' and future patients' lives).

That's what you need to do, too.

If you keep focusing on questions and fears like...

- *"Why are they getting pregnant and not me?"*
- *"Why is this happening to ME?"*
- *"Why is it so unfair?"*
- *"Will I die alone?"*
- *"Am I going to be lonely forever?"*
- *"Is my partner going to leave me?"*

...the fears are only going to get bigger. They're only going to GROW.

Those are big monsters to contend with day in and day out.

Follow what I teach you in the book, and you're going to very easily and naturally start to shift your focus away from these fears and onto the things you *are* able to control.

And in doing so the overwhelm will start to naturally fade away. You'll start to see positive changes taking root in all areas of your life, and as you do you're going to gain more and more confidence.

The Circle Of Power

I'm really, really excited for you. I really see great things ahead for you.

Earlier in this chapter I mentioned something called "The Circle Of Pain." You're about to step out of that circle into a new one.

You're about to step into your "Circle Of Power".

That's because when you follow the path in this book you will instantly have all of what I call the Three Essential Elements Of Transformation:

1. A powerful, clear, resilient mind.
2. Simple, PROVEN, non-overwhelming action steps.
3. A supportive, encouraging community of others who are not only on the fertility journey like you, but who are also approaching the journey in the unique and powerful way this book teaches.

If you will join me on this path and do the work, *I absolutely promise you this*:

You will get your power back, you will get your confidence back. You WILL get YOURSELF back.

And I don't care what anybody else says… THAT is the most direct and powerful way to facilitate the emergence of that PERFECT EGG that will become your beautiful baby. Because joy, purpose, and courage are the core of the life-creating ability you already embody.

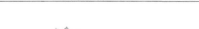

Step into a circle of support with people who are on the same journey as you… Join **Axelrad Clinic Academy** and inside you'll find a link to a special online group exclusively for readers of this book.

Visit https://axelradclinic.com/awaken to sign up now.

Chapter 4 - The Seven Core Promises

What I teach in this book is easy to do, but you must be committed to it. You can't just try a couple of things here and there and expect it to work.

In fact, it's your *commitment* to the various methods and really your ability to keep it simple that gives the teachings in this book so much power.

So, in the end you must be accountable to yourself. Only you can do this.

Nobody can do it for you and I strongly recommend that you stop waiting for buy in from anyone else.

I see a lot of people who get frustrated that their partner isn't getting on a better track with them. Or they talk about it with their friends and family members and they get negative feedback - not out of spite - just due to a lack of understanding.

You see nobody's going to really understand where you're at and what you're going through, except for a select group of people who are in a similar place spiritually and emotionally. Or people like me who have been on the front lines helping thousands find their way out.

So, you've really got to make this just about you. You've got to own this completely.

I'm not saying you should leave your partner or anything like that, or that you should isolate yourself from your family.

Of course, there are people out there - and some of them may be close to you - who unconsciously (and sometimes consciously) - create a toxic emotional environment for you.

Sometimes it's their behavior that creates friction or just doesn't mesh with you the right way. The main thing is to immediately move past blame or trying to fix it and just get to work on doing what you need to do.

You might have to distance yourself a little, or more than a little, just for your own sanity and there's no point feeling guilty about it. It's nothing personal.

Do what you need to do for yourself and don't wait for anyone to agree with you or give you their blessing. Again, you're stepping back into your power. Claim it.

And, whatever you do, don't get confused thinking that you are taking someone else's power away by claiming yours. Quite the opposite.

By claiming and embodying your own power you become a role model for others. You empower them.

So you've got to commit and go all in on this. And I've found the most effective way to do this is to make some promises to yourself.

Now look, here's where we need to stop for just one second. I want to make something very clear.

You're going to break these promises. Just go into it knowing this.

Nobody's perfect, including you. Remember we started this off with a commitment to love yourself unconditionally.

So when you "mess up" I want you to be gentle with yourself, be kind to yourself, and just be matter-of-fact about it. Forgive yourself and get right back to work.

OK so let's go ahead and learn the 7 promises, with a promise that you're going to do your best to fulfill them while being gentle and kind with yourself.

Promise #1 - Complete Ownership

I touched on this earlier - the previous chapter, in fact. You're going to take complete ownership of everything. Full responsibility for yourself.

This means you own your shit. If you feel stressed, it's because you're creating it. Things aren't stressing you out. YOU are.

It also means you don't own other people's shit. In other words, if someone else is stressing out it's because THEY'RE creating it.

It's really that simple. Again, don't make it complicated.

This also means you're not expecting anyone to come save you. You're going to be proactive and stay focused on taking the steps you need to take.

And it's important to understand complete ownership doesn't mean complete isolation. It includes owning up to the fact that there's no shame in asking for help. You haven't failed by not doing it all on your own. In fact, you are shirking your responsibility by not reaching out for help when you need it.

You must speak up if you need help.

Promise #2 - Relentless Forward Vision

This one's about something we in Texas call "staying in your lane".

I see this all the time and, of course, have done this myself. You keep looking around at all the pregnant women or women with babies around you, wondering what's different about them, endlessly making comparisons and trying to figure out why they have a baby and you don't.

Here's the thing. You can never be anyone but you. You'll never have someone else's life. It's absolutely 100% impossible, I guarantee you that.

So, you are literally throwing away your time and energy focusing on this. It's time to bring your attention back home and stay focused on what you're doing.

One of the reasons why I started off with telling you about reclaiming your power is that when you love yourself unconditionally it's a lot easier to keep this promise. It's a lot easier to feel content with who you are and being on your path vs always comparing yourself to everyone else.

A good analogy for this is something we call "rubbernecking" down here in Texas.

Rubbernecking is when there's an accident or something happening on the other side of the road but everybody starts slowing down to look and gawk. Next thing you know, your side of the road is all backed up too, even though the road is completely clear.

Comparing yourself to others is like this. It only slows you down. It causes you to take your eye off the road you're on.

Now, this does not mean you stop looking for mentors and good advice. It doesn't mean you have to figure it all out yourself. It just means you're going to keep your vision in front of you and keep taking that *one, next* step.

One more thing about this. Relentless forward focus also means you stop dwelling on the past.

Just like you can never be anybody else, you can't go back and change what happened. Obsessing over what "could have" or "should have" been is just as useless as wishing you could have someone else's life. It's a complete waste of time.

Make peace with your past by forgiving yourself and others and moving on.

Seriously, that's all you must do. Keep it simple. Forgive, be yourself, and don't dwell on past "mistakes".

Promise #3 - Track Less, Trust More

You'll find all kinds of people who recommend that you track your cycle, your temps, your this and that. And, you'll find more and more gadgets and apps to help you do it.

I'm not saying stop tracking altogether. Of course, if you want to stop tracking completely then by all means please do.

I'm just saying that I often see people track as a *substitute* for trust.

Remember the story of the seed? The seed didn't track anything. The seed just grew because that's what seeds do.

When you follow this "Awakening The Seed" method, you truly do align yourself with nature. You don't have to micromanage anything. You become like the seed - you just automatically manifest your potential.

Tracking is good for gathering data to analyze later. But most people do what I call "bare-knuckles" tracking meaning they freak out the second they notice one data point being off.

Maybe it's a low temperature, maybe it's a positive ovulation kit that's a couple of days later than "normal".

Whatever it is (and the more you're tracking, the more there is), as soon as something is "off" there is a virtual panic.

It's simply not helpful at all.

I recommend you track your cervical fluid and use an old-school ovulation test (not the electronic ones). I find this to be the most accurate and least stress-prone way for my patients to pinpoint ovulation.

Of course, if you want to just forget about tracking and just be intimate every 2-3 days, to me that's ideal, honestly. It's the proverbial "easy button" approach because you'll end up having intercourse frequently enough to cover your "fertile window" without having to worry about it.

I'm not going to get too deep into intimacy and relationships in this book. What I often see with my patients is that when they change their story, reclaim their power, and start living these promises, they start to naturally open back up to more intimacy.

If, after a few weeks doing this work, you aren't noticing any improvement in your intimacy don't panic. Be patient and give it a little more time.

You'll know if or when it's time to bring it up with your partner and seek help if you both agree to it.

Promise #4 - Follow The Plan And Take Action

I've seen quite a few people in my day who have probably done enough research on their own to deserve a PhD in Reproductive Endocrinology.

Seriously.

There are patients out there - and you might be one of them - who have as much if not more information in their heads than most doctors.

There's an old adage that "knowledge is power". In this case, trying to get pregnant, I'm just going to flat out say the amount of knowledge you have is not correlated to your power to conceive.

Not that learning some things about how to better care for your body (which I'm going to teach you), or techniques to improve circulation to your reproductive organs (which I'll also teach you), or herbs that can help speed your path to getting pregnant (yes, I'll teach you that, too) can't help.

Those things can be helpful. Very helpful. But, you must do them. Let action, not thought, be your proving ground.

Incessant research is another reflection of fear and lack of trust.

I told you the story of the seed, which (hopefully at this point) we both agree is true. The seed just DOES it.

Just like rain fell before the science of meteorology explained the mechanism, the process of conception, gestation, and birth existed and worked perfectly long before we understood them from a scientific perspective.

And, even though we now understand the mechanism of rainfall we still can't make it rain whenever we want to. So it is with fertility. We can't just "manufacture" babies on demand.

The quality we call "fertility", like rain, is just a part of nature and while there are ways to help it, in the end nature still has to do 99.9999999% of it.

So rather than theorize and pontificate and speculate, I highly recommend you get busy aligning yourself with nature through clear, consistent action like what I am teaching in this book.

I know there's a part of you that doesn't want to believe me because you feel betrayed. You were told to wait, to control your fertility and not have kids until you were ready. You were told the second you came into contact with a drop of unprotected semen you would be pregnant. And that story turned out to be wrong for you.

Then your friends may have given you advice that turned out unhelpful, and you may have even been through fertility treatment by now with no luck.

But just give this a chance to work. This is different. I'm telling you I've seen this work over and over and over again (like 2000+ times as of this writing).

Just start today and take action every day. Start with The Three Foundations which I'll discuss in the next chapter. Really do them all and do them every day.

But, not until you finish this chapter! ;-)

Promise #5 - Stay In Your Power

A major cornerstone of "Awakening The Seed", as you've probably noticed, is you reclaiming your power over your heart, your stress, and your story.

I want you to promise me you'll do your best every day to stay there.

It's easy to practice this for a few days or weeks, get some really great results, then slack off.

Reclaiming your power, your desire, and your story must be a daily commitment. Even on "good" days you need to keep doing it.

The momentum you get from daily practice is beyond anything you can imagine.

Nature flows in patterns. Day and night, the four seasons, the lunar cycle - these are well established and predictable patterns.

You want to make your new-found skill in storytelling, self-nurturing, and mindfulness as automatic and reliable as the sunrise. Daily practice is the key here.

If you're having a "bad" day (i.e. losing track of your story, beating yourself up again, forgetting your role as creator) just keep working on it. As soon as you realize you're forgetting to practice, just jump back into it right away.

Jump back into it with no worries, no judgment or regret. Don't start beating yourself up for one millisecond once you realize you've lost track.

Remember - keep your vision in front of you at all times.

Promise #6 - Be Relentlessly Loving And Kind To Yourself

One of the biggest and most devastating traps is to be hard on yourself or beat yourself up for this.

If you're like me, you couldn't do calculus when you were in the first grade…

The best, most revered calculus professor on Earth could have stood in front of you, screamed it at you, made you read it over and over and over and you never would have learned it. Why?

Because you simply weren't at a stage of development where you could process the information. Your brain literally could not process the information at that point in your life.

Now, let me ask you this - are you going to call yourself stupid or beat the hell out of yourself because you couldn't learn calculus in the first grade?

Of course not. So, why are you beating yourself up now? Why are you taking your situation as punishment or as an opportunity to blame yourself and second guess yourself?

In the chapter about Awakening The Seed I showed you how to open your heart to unconditional love for yourself. To be your own advocate and to stop waiting for the world to give you unconditional love.

So, you just have to do it.

Unconditional love isn't about REASONS. It's not about achievement or social status or income or whether you've succeeded at this or that or having a baby or whatever.

You choose to love yourself right now, no questions asked.

This promise goes with all the other promises but particularly the promise of relentless forward focus. You're going to stop looking back, wondering about all the what ifs, the forks in the road, the people who did this or that to you. You're going to stay right here, in the present, and love yourself with all your heart FIRST.

There's no more bargaining, no more logic, no more judgment. No more "I deserve this" or "it's not meant to be" or "I'm not fit to be a mother" or whatever else you might be feeling in the deep dark recesses. Those things bubble up and give you a lot of grief.

When they bubble up you absolutely must choose to love yourself in that moment. Remember you're creating the fear, guilt, shame, frustration - and then create peace and joy by loving yourself anyway.

Next chapter's "Awakening The Seed" exercise will help you cultivate and develop this new habit of showing kindness and mercy towards yourself with an open heart. It's something we all struggle with, and this practice - done faithfully - ends that struggle.

Promise #7 - Stop Seeking To Be Understood

I'm going to tell you something now that might be a shock. But, it's something you absolutely need to know.

99% of people will ever truly understand the pain you're feeling around this situation.

True, your partner is invested in it. Your parents, family, and friends are also pulling for you.

But they can never fully understand what YOU are going through right now.

YOU are the one who is feeling the pain, you are the one who must find your way out.

You don't need buy in from anyone else, you don't need anyone else to understand the pain you're in, and the more you look around for sympathy or empathy, the more you're just wasting time, honestly.

Here's the deal - there are a lot of people out there who thrive on recruiting others into their pain. Whether it's their indignation at perceived mistreatment by others, or their dislike for the boss, or their family problems, there are just some people that must share it with as many who will listen because they need the validation.

I want you to validate YOURSELF. Hell yes this hurts, hell yes it's not where you imagined you'd be.

And, hell yes, you're going to do something about it. You're going to stop talking about it and do something about it.

Now, I'm not advocating that you isolate yourself. You absolutely need what I call a "Circle Of Power" that you can lean on. You absolutely need to reach out to and be in contact with others who are going through this.

But, only in VERY RARE cases are those people in your circle of friends and family.

Awakening The Seed is a different kind of method for women trying to conceive. It's not a bunch of facts and figures. It's not fear-based and it's not confusing. It's simple and it's about self-empowerment in every way possible.

I truly believe *Awakening The Seed* is the most effective way because when I started teaching this to my patients they started getting pregnant and having babies much more often. In fact, my patients doing IVF started having over 70% success rate and my non-IVF patients around 50%.

That's because it is a way of harnessing nature's power - the power that's right here, this moment, inside you.

But, what you must understand is not everybody wants to own their power. In fact, most people want to continue "the blame and shame game" to explain why they have the problems they have. They're more interested in pointing fingers than taking ownership. They're always going to shift blame to circumstances, other people, or themselves.

Blame implies guilt which implies judgment. Blame is about "right and wrong" or "good and bad". With *Awakening The Seed* we're stepping out of that game and moving forward with relentless, ruthless unconditional love for ourselves and our lives.

It's critical that you surround yourself with others who want the same thing.

Trust me, just by connecting with them, you will accelerate your path to freedom from pain, anxiety, and overwhelm and - when you are on that path - you are on a VERY direct path to getting pregnant.

Chapter 5 - How To Re-Awaken Your Innate Ability To Create Life

I know you're probably wondering when I'm going to get to all the diet tips and supplements and exercise advice and all that.

Don't worry I've got that stuff coming in Part Two of the book (and of course, you're free to skip ahead if you like).

But I think it's crucial that we first go over the stuff nobody else tells you or teaches you - at least not in the way you're about to learn it here.

You've probably - no, I'll bet you've almost certainly - done your research on diet tips and supplements and read all the "10 ways to…" and "21 things you should never..." blog posts by the self-styled experts on these matters.

You've probably even tried a bunch of the things they recommended, too. Yet, here we are.

So, if I just started spouting off all my little "diet tricks" and "magic supplements" I'd just be giving you more of the same - which hasn't exactly worked out to this point.

What I've discovered working with thousands of people one-on-one is that the pills and procedures - the supplements, herbs, acupuncture, and all that stuff - are incredible tools that can facilitate change in the body.

But, there is no pill or procedure to override the often toxic effects of a self-defeating, over-stressed, anxiety-ridden mind. There's not a drug, herb, food, surgery, acupuncture point, or anything else that's going to overcome that.

I've seen people who've done 5, 7, even 10+ rounds of IVF. Nobody could explain why they weren't getting pregnant.

All the best pills, supplements, drugs, procedures… Everything was brought to bear. Yet, nothing.

And, in a good number of these cases I've personally witnessed the most simple shifts in thought and feeling be the catalyst that brings everything together and creates the right conditions for pregnancy to finally take root.

With the proper mindset you no longer struggle. You're not swimming against the current anymore.

You suddenly start to just "know" what you need to do next. There's no more hand-wringing worry or brain-melting online research.

Your way forward becomes crystal clear, almost like somebody suddenly handed you a map.

Which is what happens when you tap into Seed Intelligence. You simply KNOW what to do because you have uncovered the source map within yourself.

That's why I call this first exercise "Awakening The Seed." And it's for sure the most important thing you need to be doing right now if you want to end the anxiety and overwhelm that has taken over your life.

And, good news, it's a lot easier than you think. In fact, you already know how to do it.

At first it might feel a little strange because it's been a long time since you did it. But, you still remember. You haven't forgotten. It's like the proverbial "riding a bike." Except you learned this before you were even born.

Here's how you do it:

Ruthlessly, unapologetically love yourself. Completely. Unconditionally. RELENTLESSLY.

Just like you love your future child.

The world can be a very unkind place. In fact, I think it's safe to say that it IS a very unkind place in many, many ways.

But I believe we created it that way to drive ourselves to look inward for refuge. We created it that way to force us to look within and eventually come back home to ourselves.

There is no greater power than "Unconditional Self-Directed Loving-Kindness". Period. Nothing more powerful.

And, while you may think this has nothing to do with getting pregnant, I assure you it has EVERYTHING to do with it.

There's a reason adoption paperwork routinely queries prospective adoptive parents as to whether they're adopting because they think it will help them get pregnant.

It's because so many people actually DO get pregnant after adopting.

I'm not saying everyone does, but it happens often enough to where it's a standard question on adoption applications, to make sure you're adopting for the right reasons.

People will say that the reason this happens - people getting pregnant after adopting - is because they stop thinking about it and relax.

But I disagree completely.

Anyone with a newborn will tell you the experience is anything BUT relaxing and stress-free. It's a huge learning curve (especially for first-time parents) coupled with sleepless nights, adjusting to an entirely new relationship dynamic (two's company, three's a crowd, right?), and a whole new set of "problems" arises like…

"Where is junior going to school? Who is going to be the pediatrician? How much screen time is too much?"

So, in my view the spontaneous pregnancies after adopting is not because the adoptive parents relax and stop thinking about it.

It's that once they have the baby (or sometimes even just KNOWING they're going to have a baby) they feel a deep, profound, unconditional love they were unable to feel without the baby there.

You see, in the end, this is why you really want a baby. You may think it's for all these other more practical (or not-so-practical) reasons.

But when it comes down to it, you want to remember who YOU are. You want to feel the joy of unconditional love you once felt for yourself.

Babies naturally bring that out in all of us because they remind us of where we came from - when we were naturally clear-minded, innocent, and full of joy and love.

It's why baby pictures get 10,000 likes on social media and why even the most sullen, sad, or angry person suddenly makes goo-goo sounds and baby-talk when they see one.

So, if the most important key to this process is to reconnect with that simple joy of unconditional love, what I want to ask you is, "What the heck are you waiting for?"

Reclaim your power right here, right now. Experience that unconditional love by giving it back to yourself via the "Awakening The Seed" exercise.

There are a few rules to this exercise:

1. Be loving, kind, and supportive always.
2. Be yourself.
3. Allow the child to be him/herself.
4. Listen and pay attention to the dialogue, if any.

Here are the steps:

1. Close your eyes, take 10 very slow, relaxed, deep breaths. Don't force it. And breathe into your belly.
2. Now, visualize yourself as a child. I want you to see the child in a scene or setting. They don't know you're there. They're busy doing something.
3. Observe your child self. What is s/he wearing? What is s/he doing? Where is s/he? Is there anyone else there? What's going on?
4. Now, after some time, I want you to imagine that your child self turns and sees you.

114

5. You make eye contact. It is a HAPPY moment. The child is happy to see you, and you are happy to see the child.

6. Now, approach the child, offer a hug. Take the child's hand and go somewhere safe. Whatever that is for you.

7. Sit with the child in this safe place.

8. Tell the child that you love them completely and unconditionally, and you will always be there for them. That you are here now, and you will never, ever go away again. Feel that the child believes you and trusts you. You are making a sacred promise.

9. If the child says anything to you, listen and make note. You can answer but make sure you answer from a place of kindness and not judgment – reaffirm your support and love. What the child says may make sense, it may not.

10. Whatever they say, REMEMBER IT. You're going to write it down later.

11. Now, spend a little more time with the child. Just do whatever you feel like – there's no right or wrong way to do this. You might have a conversation, or play, or just sit and hold the child. Whatever you like.

12. When you are ready, tell the child it is time for you to go. But, promise them you'll be back, and you are going to be with them no matter what, and if they need anything to let you know and you'll be back to spend time with them again.

13. Take a few more deep breaths and open your eyes.

14. Now take out a notebook or your computer and write down what happened.

15. Be as detailed as possible within the time you have. Make sure, if nothing else, that you write down what the child said when you asked what you could do to help them.

This exercise can bring up some strong emotions. But, you will be OK. Don't worry. Just keep focusing on sending love and kindness to this beautiful child part of yourself.

You'll find an audio track to guide you through this, and the other meditations and visualizations in this book, in the always free **Axelrad Clinic Academy**.
Visit https://axelradclinic.com/awaken to sign up now.

Chapter 6 - How To Rediscover And Reawaken Your Massive Creative Potential

The next critical step on this journey, as I alluded to before, is for you to make a very important and crucial choice.

Up until now, you've had a particular story. It started off with you pretty much just getting pregnant, having your baby and moving forward from there. It was a simple, innocent, clear story.

But, for whatever reason, that story hasn't worked out. I can't tell you why and there's no sense beating your head against the wall trying to figure it out at this point.

The main thing is that, at this point, your story has likely become a very, very painful one.

All of us are storytellers. In fact, I believe it's what makes us human, as opposed to animals or plants. We tell stories - and we're really good at it.

But it's also our ability to tell stories that gets us into trouble. That's because we can make up some really crazy and strange stories that cause things like arguments, hurt feelings, and even wars.

In fact, I truly believe that all pain and suffering in the human realm comes from stories that reflect something other than our true nature, which is limitless and unconditional joy and love.

The cool thing here is that you have free will. At any time, you can choose to tell yourself a new story. You don't have to keep living in the scary, overwhelming, painful story you may be living in now.

You can wake up from that and create a new story and, by doing so, completely change your state of being.

Notice what I said there. It was very intentional. I said state of *being* not just state of *mind*.

That's because EVERYTHING will change in very profound ways that support your fertility. Not only your thoughts, actions, and feelings, but even the structure, composition, and function of the cells, organs, and tissues that make up your body.

Let me illustrate.

The Raw Biological Power Of The Stories We Tell Ourselves

Imagine I sit you down in a movie theater and I hook you up to a super-high-tech Bluetooth monitoring device that sends real-time measurements to my laptop screen of your brain waves, circulation, blood pressure, cardiac electrical waves, every hormone and neurotransmitter, and just about every other possible biochemical, electrical, and functional measurement of your body.

I step out, and the theater goes dark as I start playing a scary movie on the movie screen in front of you. Something like one of those thrillers where there's ten people in a remote cabin out in the woods by a lake and some crazed lunatic is killing everyone off one by one. Lots of suspense, gore, and startling moments.

Without fail (unless you're a highly-trained Zen monk) the numbers and graphs on my laptop for heart rate, blood pressure, electrical activity of your heart & brain, hormones, neurotransmitters - will be pure chaos.

Brain waves... chaos.

Heart pulses... rapid and irregular.

Blood pressure... all over the place.

Blood oxygen... low.

Capillaries... constricted.

See where I'm going here...??

And let's not even talk about how the stress hormones like cortisol and prolactin are climbing, while calming hormones like serotonin and dopamine and endorphin are declining.

Oxidative stress is higher, and the natural antioxidant function of your body is severely challenged because of the increased stress on all cells and tissues.

So, what's happening here?

Well, in terms of your environment... NOTHING.

You're simply watching a movie, a *story*, that is not really happening. Just a bunch of images and sounds on a screen. Actors pretending. A total farce.

But the chaotic, constricted biological state I just described?

That is as real as it gets.

So, I turn off the scary movie and give you a minute to rest. Then, I start playing a romantic comedy. It's a feel-good story about two people who were best friends since grade school and when they grow up they realize that they're really in love with each other. And, of course, they live this amazing life and are forever happy and, even when times get tough, their love sees them through to the end.

How do you think those readings on my screen are looking now?

- The brain and cardiac waves are smooth and calm.
- The circulation, respiration and blood pressure relaxed and even.
- And, the blood is loaded with calming, feel-good hormones and neurotransmitters: endorphins, dopamine, and serotonin.
- Oxidative stress is scarcely present.
- Capillaries are wide open, and every cell is getting all the nutrients and oxygen (aka "life") it needs in abundance.

And the only difference is… you guessed it… THE STORY ON THE SCREEN.

The love story I'm showing you now is no more "real" than the scary one I was showing you before. Neither are happening. Nobody's really falling in love, and nobody's really trapped in a cabin in the woods with a crazed lunatic hiding in the basement.

I know what you're thinking. "Sure Chris, but those are movies, and this is my life. The movies aren't real, but this is. "

True enough.

Except this: *All those images in your mind depicting how miserable you're going to be, how there's no hope, how you're not going to have a legacy, how you're going to die alone, how your partner is going to leave you or whatever other thing you're telling yourself - none of that is real, either.*

None of it has happened or is happening. You're literally making it all up. Like the horror movie above, it's a STORY playing on the movie screen of your mind.

And, despite what anyone has told you to the contrary, you absolutely have the power to press STOP on that movie, and completely replace it with a love story.

In fact, if you've already practiced "Awakening The Seed", you've already taken the most powerful step possible in that direction. So, congratulations! (And, if you haven't practiced it yet, now would be a great time to go back and do it. ;-)).

Taking ownership of the imagery and language you are projecting into your mind is, in my view, *the* most powerful thing a human being can do because by doing so you gain the power to literally reconfigure your biology.

Remember the two movies we just showed you, and your two very different biological responses to those movies?

We're going to take charge of the imagery and language inside your mind, and by doing so we're going to initiate powerful shifts in your cells, tissues, organs, and hormones - INCLUDING your FSH, LH, follicles, eggs, uterus, and everything else.

And, on top of this… you're going to find these simple daily mindset rituals make the dietary and lifestyle changes we will discuss in Part Two 100x easier to incorporate.

And here's why this will work so well for you:

Your subconscious mind will believe whatever you keep telling it.

It's how hypnosis works. It's how repetition and practice help us learn new skills like playing a musical instrument or typing or driving until they become - so to speak - *automatic*.

121

So, by committing to practice these simple mindset rituals you'll essentially be learning how to generate a state of fertility in your body... *on autopilot*. It will be easy, effortless, and happening all the time, every day.

I truly believe this is the key to why so many of my patients who follow this process end up having a baby, and rarely have problems when it comes time to have their next 1, 2, or more children.

It's because they have accessed and reconfigured the source code of life-creation to work in their favor. Literally.

But this does require you to be diligent and spend the 5-10 minutes a day required for it to work, even when you think it might not be working.

I want you to think about a medication. You swallow the pill, then you wait for your body to respond. You don't have to "think your way" into the response to the medicine - deciding how your stomach will dissolve it, or how your liver will metabolize it, or which receptors it will activate on which cells or how your body will excrete it.

Your body is so incredibly intelligent and has so much wisdom and power embedded within that it just does all that, on its own, without a single conscious thought on your part.

Now, we know with medications sometimes it may take days or weeks for the full effects to kick in. And, there may be days early on where you begin to wonder if it will ever work. But, if you want the result badly enough, you'll keep swallowing the pill every day until the effects are real.

Your *mind* works the exact same way, but with words and stories.

You feed yourself a thought, a belief, or a perspective, and your subconscious mind digests it, metabolizes it, incorporates it and RESPONDS to it (again, remember the response to the two different movies above).

Sometimes the results aren't immediately apparent, and it's then that the scared, worried, frustrated part of ourselves will think, "Oh, this is total BS. It's not going to do anything…" And, many give up because of this.

I have two words for you: DON'T LISTEN.

Keep "swallowing" that mental "pill" over and over, day in and day out, and I PROMISE that within 3-5 days you will notice changes in your overall mood, your level of focus, and - most importantly - your energy level.

That's because - as I said above - these words, these images, and these breathing techniques change the structure of your subconscious mind, just like eating clean, low-carb, nutrient-dense food leads to weight loss and stronger body function.

Essentially, everything in Part One here is about the most important food of all that nobody else thinks about: The words and images you continually "consume" inside your mind.

And, once you shift the habitual language and imagery of your subconscious mind the results (i.e. you getting pregnant) can be VERY, VERY FAST.

Why?

So many of my patients who now have babies had been "trying to conceive" for 2, 3, even 5 years before working with me and within 3-6 months fell pregnant.

To me, that means all along they were missing the mark by millimeters, not miles. Let me illustrate.

If we water a plant just enough every day, it will survive but it will not thrive.

We can water that plant the same way for 2, 3, even 5 years - giving it just enough water to get by - and the plant will still be JUST SHORT of its full potential, even though it is alive and doesn't look "unhealthy".

Yet... as soon as we give it a few extra ml of water for a week or two... BOOM. Full bloom. And we realize then that, "Oh, wow, I wasn't giving this plant all the water it needed all these years."

And, what represents "full bloom" more - from a human biological perspective - than a fertile, energy-filled egg ready to grow into a baby?

If there's a better example, I can't think of it.

Let me warn you again about a common pitfall. And this is important, so pay attention:

When you commit to changing your story the way I'm going to teach you here in a minute, a part of you is going to push back and tell you it's BS.

Totally natural. In fact, that push-back is a sign that it's WORKING. Why?

Because there's a part of yourself (called ego) that LOVES your old story. It wants to stay with the familiar. It perceives change as a threat - even if that means letting go of anxiety, worry, doubt, frustration, sadness.

So, that "this is BS" push-back is a sign your ego KNOWS this stuff is going to work (aka it's going to result in you replacing that old story with a new, more powerful story that WILL facilitate fertility-positive shifts in your body).

And, this is why the "Awakening The Seed" process begins with a commitment to LOVE that part of yourself that is scared, afraid, and needs your nurturing, loving care.

Bottom line is this: I *assure* you, if you keep "swallowing the pill", your new story will sink into your subconscious mind and, like a drug, it will start to have that profoundly positive impact on your egg quality and every single other aspect of your ability to conceive and give birth to your baby.

And all of it will happen literally on autopilot, without any extra effort.

The key, however, is you must keep "swallowing the medicine" (i.e. telling the story to yourself) to give it time to work.

Nobody would ever expect to heal from a long-standing health issue simply by taking one single pill one time. It just doesn't happen.

The same holds true for the practice of "Intentional Storytelling", which we're about to learn in a minute. You've got to commit to taking the medicine regularly if you expect it to work.

The Miracle Of Seed Intelligence

Earlier I mentioned that you already contain the exact blueprint for how you're going to overcome this. The entire answer lies within you.

I also told you a story about a seedling that takes root and grows simply by trusting the wisdom it already embodies.

I call this "The story of the seed". And it goes like this:

1. A seed falls on the ground.
2. It sinks into the soil and as soon as it contacts the water and soil...
3. It awakens with life and starts to grow.
4. It already knows which way is up and which way is down.
5. It already knows exactly what it is supposed to do.
6. It instinctively sends its roots downward into the earth and reaches its leaves and branches up towards the light of the sun.
7. It just keeps growing and growing - encountering and adapting to all sorts of difficulties along the way with silent, unrelenting grace and resilience - until, one day, it's a beautiful, majestic, fully grown tree.
8. The seed didn't have to do anything special. It simply did what nature guided it to do. It contained the entire blueprint from the beginning.

Now, don't make it complicated. Don't think too hard about this. It's a very simple story.

And, I absolutely promise, it's your story.

How do I know this? Because you and I both started as seeds (eggs and sperm) and somehow ended up as these complete human beings with all our incredibly intelligent cells and organs, able to think and feel and dream and love.

Do you realize the power in that?

That's how I see all the people I work with. I see them as magnificent embodiments of nature's unfathomable creative power.

And, that's how I see you.

You may have forgotten this story, but now you remember.

And you and I both know beyond any doubt that this story is true.

The question is, are you going to keep telling yourself that other story. You know, the one where you've lost your power and there's little hope you'll ever be happy?

Or, are you going to stop telling that lie to yourself and start telling a story that reflects your true brilliance and your present and real capacity to create new life right here, right now?

The choice is always yours. And I know you will make the best one for you.

I've created a simple exercise to help you clarify and concentrate your story around having a baby. By doing so, you'll be generating a powerful mental and emotional center around which all your efforts will unify.

Remember my principle of "Unification" above? There's nothing more powerful for concentrating creative energy and guiding your cells and biology into a more open, fertile state.

True, the pills, procedures, and practices are important. They're a part of the equation just like we must eat AND breathe.

But the force that keeps us on track, more than anything else, is the story we're telling ourselves about the past, present, and future.

Own Your Story

I have a little exercise for you now. It's simple, and I don't want you to make it complicated. I call it "Own Your Story" and its designed to help you focus your desire like a laser beam.

Again... desire is the most powerful force for creating change. In fact, it is really the *only* change-making force.

And stories are the most powerful tools we must concentrate our desire to shape not only our destiny, but also our physiology and biology.

Think about it: You watch a scary movie and your heart races and your adrenaline pumps. You watch a love story and your heart soars, and you're loaded with endorphins.

We are telling ourselves stories all the time whether consciously or subconsciously. Some of the stories are happy, some are sad. Some are angry, some are compassionate. Some are about us as victims, others about us as perpetrators, etc.

The point is that they're all just *stories*. If you choose to tell yourself a sad story about what's happening or what might happen or even what has happened, it's just your *story* about it. That's it. There's no reality to it. Someone else might look at the same situation and see victory, while another sees a disaster.

That's what's happening in your subconscious mind, 24 hours a day.

So, what you must do is decide how you're going to answer this simple question: *"What's my story?"*

Because your story is going to set your physiological foundation more than you realize.

In fact, one of the great secrets of life is that our bodies are strongly influenced (some would say they're literally shaped) by stories. Regardless of what you believe, I can tell you without a doubt that the stories you accept and repeat have a profound influence on every cell in your body.

See for yourself by practicing the exercise below for at least 7 days in a row.

1. Get out a notebook or journal and a pen.
2. Close your eyes, take a few deep, relaxed breaths, and bring to mind your current story about yourself and how you're expecting this "fertility journey" you're on to work out. Just be brutally honest with yourself - nobody's watching and nobody's grading you.
3. Now, write that story down – summarize it in two or three paragraphs.
4. Now, close your eyes, take a few deep breaths again, and visualize the most hopeful, joyful, "positive" story you can about your future as a mother, and the journey to that day when you give birth to your baby.

5. Really let yourself visualize it. Don't hold back. Make it as uplifting and inspiring as you can – even if you don't believe it at all (and your subconscious will try to talk you out of it, so just ignore any background "this-is-BS" kind of feelings).
6. Now write that story. Again – summarize and hit the main points.
7. Close the notebook or journal.

Next, all you must do is simply read your positive story at least 2x a day – for instance in the morning and before bed. *Don't miss one day.*

At the end of 7 days make some notes on the page underneath your new, positive story, about the changes you've noticed. And, if you want, go ahead and repeat the exercise again to see how your stories have changed. Or, just stay with the one you have for now and keep going. Trust me, you'll know what to do.

You'll find an audio track to guide you through this, and the other meditations and visualizations in this book, in the always free
Axelrad Clinic Academy.
Visit https://axelradclinic.com/awaken to sign up now.

If you're still reading, congratulations. You've made a great decision.

Not only have you just learned one of the most important techniques for using your consciousness to shift the function of your hormones, you're about to learn a life-changing technique that - in my experience helping 2000+ women just like you to overcome their own obstacles to having their babies - is the fastest and most effective way to boost your   fertility.

I call it "Transforming Stress Into Fertility" and it can truly set you on a whole new course almost instantly.

So, let's go to the next chapter where I'll teach you exactly how to do it.

Chapter 7 - Why Stress Isn't The Problem - And What IS

You see, there was a moment, an instant, when you decided to come into this world. When you asked yourself, "Do I want to live? Do I want to enter the proving grounds of earth and experience the ups and downs and victories and defeats that life on earth inevitably requires?"

And - obviously - you said "yes."

OK, not just "yes." But, "YES!"

We call that moment your first heartbeat. In that moment you were fully aware of your power and you fully embraced it.

Prior to that, your entire body was one cell, then two, then four, then eight, then thousands, then millions and billions and trillions.

Science has tried for decades to understand exactly how you did that.

It's still a complete mystery.

What science *has* figured out is that - via stem cells - you create all your organs and cells and all the root tissues to support you on your journey within the first 10 weeks of your existence.

And around 4 weeks into that process, just 4 weeks after your entire body was just one cell, you created your first heartbeat.

Even though your organs and tissues were far from fully developed, you were ready.

You didn't need to "know" exactly how the story ends before you said YES. You simply did it. You went for it because you knew how powerful you were.

And, if you're like most, along the road of life you forgot about that incredible creative power you embody.

Today is the day you're going to reclaim it, should you choose. And, like I said, it's not hard. In fact, you already know how to do it.

We've talked about your story - the key to you waking up. And, we've talked about your desire for unconditional love and your ability to express it here and now, which continually guides your Seed Intelligence and helps you to overcome the anxiety, worry, frustration, and other painful emotions you feel.

Now, we're going to begin to regain our power over those emotional states which, as I pointed out earlier, interfere with the signals that guide our body's natural Seed Intelligence - much like storms interfere with radio and satellite transmissions.

To regain our power, we're going to use a special technique I developed that anyone can do. It's a simple, daily practice that very rapidly taps you back into the immense power you must shape your destiny - including having your baby.

Before I get to that though I want to be clear on what I'm talking about when I refer to "stress."

The kind of stress I'm talking about here is the common definition - meaning unpleasant feelings and thoughts like fear, anger, shame, guilt, grief, sadness, frustration, and others.

However, I want to be crystal clear - stress is more than just unpleasant feelings. There are many, many "hidden" stressors that we will address later in the book, including:

- Lack of sleep, restless sleep, and arrhythmic sleep patterns.
- Chronic, low-grade dehydration.
- Metabolic instability due to eating out of sync with hormonal rhythms.
- Unresolved, chronic, low-grade inflammation.
- Lack of blood flow to critical cells and tissues which deprives them of oxygen, nutrients, and hormones.

All the above states are incredibly stressful for your cells, organs, and tissues as they constantly, faithfully adapt to the lack of rest, lack of nutrients, and lack of consistency and predictability we so commonly throw at them.

The good news is that later, when we get into the incredibly simple and powerful lifestyle and diet shifts I've used with thousands of my patients to help them conceive, I'm going to teach you how to eliminate all these hidden stressors.

So, I don't want you to worry at all.

But it's critically important to help you gain the upper hand on the emotional side first. That's because if you're at the whim of these emotional states and can't sustain your focus, it doesn't matter WHAT dietary or lifestyle changes I teach you or how many acupuncture treatments you get, the positive changes and results will be less sustainable and - as a result - a LOT less reliable.

Emotional stress, like everything else, is just a form of energy. And, like all forms of energy, it moves. That's why they're called eMOTIONs.

134

Emotions themselves (even the negative ones) are natural, and we will always feel them. They only become a problem when we hold onto them instead of just feeling them and letting them go.

Imagine the sky. Some days it's clear. Other days it's cloudy. But, the air is always in motion. We know, for a fact, that if today is cloudy it will at some point clear up again. And, that if today is clear and sunny at some point it will once again rain.

We accept this as fact as "just the way nature works".

It's the same with our emotional states, but in the case of our feelings we fight these natural movements and shifts.

Whether it's anger, guilt, shame, fear, or grief - or even the positive emotions of joy, excitement, pride, and affection - the emotions themselves aren't what causes problems for us.

It's when we want them to be different or get stuck on them - and they start to overwhelm us - that things become problematic.

But there's a hidden treasure in these emotions - even the "negative ones".

I've learned how to extract this precious treasure and use it in my own life, and I've also taught my patients this same technique to dramatically boost egg quality and fertility.

See, all the overwhelm, anxiety, frustration, and other crippling emotions you are feeling right now represent a tremendous amount of energy.

And, I've discovered a technique that reclaims, refines, and redirects that energy straight into your body's fertility process - including the process of creating that perfect egg that will produce your perfect baby.

I call this technique "Transforming Stress Into Fertility" and it is one of the most - if the THE most - life-transforming things you will ever learn. Not only will it be a huge difference-maker on your fertility journey, it will be a pivotal mind shift that will improve your relationships, your mental focus and calm, and your overall quality of life.

Here's a little story to illustrate how this works:

I guarantee you the first people who found oil seeping up through the ground had no idea how much power that stinky, messy, black liquid contained.

In fact, I guarantee you they ran away from it as fast as they could. After all, unrefined crude oil is extremely toxic.

And, all those negative emotions that feel so overwhelming during times of struggle in our lives, they're a lot like that crude oil.

Stinky, messy, and unpleasant.

Which is why we react to fear, frustration, worry, overwhelm, and these other negative emotions by trying to get away from them.

After you learn how to transform this "emotional crude oil" into highly refined, joyful calm, you're going to suddenly find yourself sitting on a fertility goldmine - just like the person who first learned how to refine crude oil into gasoline, jet fuel, and other powerful energy sources.

Except their gold isn't nearly as precious as yours will be.

And here's another cool thing about this process: You don't have to go out looking for the energy because, well, you're using the emotions you already generate.

That's right. Unlike the companies drilling for oil, you don't have to go on an elaborate exploration to find the energy.

It's right here, right now. You're creating it all the time. And, this is a crucial thing to understand.

You see, all your life you've been told your stress is "out there." That things, people, circumstances, people cutting you off in traffic, long lines at the grocery store or airport, and other world events are "stressing you out".

Bottom line: That's simply not true.

Most people blame their stress on all those things because - to be completely blunt about it - they have forgotten their power and, hence, won't take responsibility for themselves.

With "Transforming Stress Into Fertility" we're going to learn to stop doing that. And it's going to set us free.

Before we get into the technique itself, let me remind you that you don't have to do ANY of this stuff perfectly for it to work. You just have to create a tiny little opening for nature to break through and create new life in you.

That's because, as I like to say, "Nature can do a hell of a lot with *good enough*."

So, the most important part is to get started and take consistent imperfect action. You'll learn as you go, trust me.

When you commit to the practice of Transforming Stress Into Fertility, you're taking full ownership of your inner space.

You'll be living my one of my most important credos:

"Own your thoughts. Own your feelings. Own your life."

When you own your thoughts, you no longer allow yourself to (erroneously) think thoughts like "that stresses me out" or "you're making me sad / angry / disappointed /etc."

- "You're stressing me out…" becomes "I'm creating stress in response to your words or behavior."
- "I'm really anxious" … becomes "I am creating anxiety."
- "Today is a stressful day…" becomes "I am generating a lot of stress today."

Do you feel the power in that?

When you shift your internal language to embrace the truth that, in fact, you are the one generating the feeling and emotion, you immediately gain complete power over them.

Why?

Because when you realize and accept that you are creating these emotions by choice (even if that is a subconscious choice), then - and *only* then - can you learn to choose new emotions.

With TSIF (Transforming Stress Into Fertility) you are accepting them as yours. With no judgment.

And, because you own it, you now have the power to transform it.

You can take that massive reserve of emotional energy locked up inside all the fear, frustration, worry, and overwhelm - that crude oil you thought was a stinky, slimy mess - and begin to literally transform it into fertile, creative energy.

And it's actually very easy to do. In fact, once you've done this a few times, you'll feel like it's completely natural.

That's because - like I said in the introduction - it *is* completely natural. You already know how to do it.

I want to stress something here: If you haven't already, it's VERY IMPORTANT that you practice the "Awakening The Seed" meditation a few times before you start doing this. And, here's why...

The technique I'm going to teach you is going to create a new level of mindfulness in you. You're going to start noticing things that you hadn't noticed before.

A lot of what you're going to notice may not be so "pretty". You might start to notice anger, impatience, low self-esteem, self-pity, self-sabotage, etc.

We've all been taught to avoid these kinds of feelings or to think that they're "bad" - or to ignore them to the point where we don't even realize we're engaging in them.

So, it's critical that you familiarize yourself with the practice of "Awakening The Seed" so you are continually cultivating unconditional love towards yourself.

That way, you will find it a LOT easier to transform all these negative emotions into positive, creative energy.

Another thing I want to make sure you understand: This is NOT a "cop out."

People have told me before that they think this technique is a way to ignore or deny feelings. This couldn't be further from the truth.

When you practice this consistently you are becoming incredibly aware of your feelings. You are bearing witness like you never have before.

But now - instead of judging yourself for them or feeling like you're, the victim and they have power over you - you are redirecting the energy of those emotions into positive, creative channels.

This opens a TREMENDOUS amount of space for your body to operate in a harmonious way. Why?

Remember in chapter two, I told you about stories. I told you about how powerful stories are in terms of how they impact your physiology.

Then, later, you envisioned and wrote your Powerful Story - the story of reaching your destiny as a mother. That's a *future* story.

"Transforming Your Stress Into Fertility" is about continually changing your *present* story - the one you tell yourself moment to

140

moment - into a story that reflects truth and concentrates your creative power.

You see, all that moment-to-moment anger, fear, guilt, regret - whatever negative emotions you repeatedly experience - these are just a result of the story you're telling yourself RIGHT NOW.

By using my TSIF technique, you're going to be continually redirecting your story and, by doing so, you're going to be continually releasing all that raw energy back into your biology which it will use to generate a more positive, creative, fertile state.

Whatever you do, though, you must promise you'll stick to it. Just keep working on it. Don't give up. Just like when you first learned how to ride a bike, you might not get the feel of it right away. It may not seem like much is happening.

So, commit to at least 3-4 days of consistent practice.

Also, once you learn this technique, you practice it continuously. There's no need to wait until you're in a quiet room sitting in lotus pose to do it. This is a "walking meditation" in that you do it as you go about your normal life.

How To Transform Stress Into Fertility

Let's go ahead and practice quick so you can see just how easy and natural this is…

1. Take a few deep breaths and let your body relax.
2. Imagine a recent situation where you were upset by something. Anything will do. Maybe someone cut you off in traffic, or someone said something that rubbed you the wrong

way, or a friend or family member told you they were pregnant.

3. Whatever it was, bring it to mind now. I want you to feel how you felt in that moment.

4. Now, just like you're rewinding a movie on your TV, rewind back to the exact moment you were triggered.

5. Imagine that instead of just reacting the way you did, you noticed those feelings coming up. You were able to notice yourself getting frustrated, annoyed, or grief-stricken.

6. You started to feel it, but instead of going with it and letting it escalate, you said (to yourself):

7. "I am feeling [name of feeling]. As the creator of this [name of feeling here], I choose to create joy and inner peace instead."

8. Then, generate that feeling of joy and inner peace, to the best of your ability. If you can't feel it, then imagine you can feel it. With time, you will start to feel it, so don't give up.

You'll find an audio track to guide you through this, and the other meditations and visualizations in this book, in the always free
Axelrad Clinic Academy.
Visit https://axelradclinic.com/awaken to sign up now.

Now, I want to point something out.

In the first sentence above, you did something very important: You named the emotion.

Naming things gives us power over them. It proves that we "see" them when we can name them.

Claiming ownership of things gives us power as well. In this case, you take responsibility for the fact that you created that feeling.

That's why the next thing you say is, "As the creator of this [name of feeling here], I choose to create joy and inner peace instead."

When you say that, I want you to feel a sense of joy and inner peace. CREATE that joy and inner peace. Do not passively wait for it to arrive.

This might feel awkward to you at first. Again, it's not like most of us are ever taught to consciously and intentionally generate emotional states.

But - trust me - you know all about how to do it.

And, the reason I want you to start out by specifically generating "joy and inner peace" is because this joyful, peaceful state is your essential nature. It's who you are at your core.

It's the source of Seed Intelligence.

So, speak it to yourself. Say you're choosing to transform that negative emotion into joy and inner peace, then DO IT.

In fact, right now, generate that sense of joy and inner peace. Right this second, just do it.

Did you feel that?

You may have felt it strongly or subtly, but I know you felt something shift.

I've seen this shift happen hundreds and hundreds of times as I've taught this method, and thousands of times myself as I've practiced it. If you give it a chance and work with it, it never fails.

And, I truly believe it's one of the most important things you can do to enhance your fertility. So, don't forget to do this as often as you possibly can. I promise it will make everything easier.

Yes, we have treatment options for people outside the Houston area to help you optimize your egg quality and get pregnant as soon as possible.

Visit https://axelradclinic.com/remote for details and availability.

Part Two
Core Daily Rituals For Optimal Egg Quality

"Water is the softest thing, yet it can penetrate mountains and earth. This shows clearly the principle of softness overcoming hardness."
- Lao Tzu

Chapter 8 - The Three Foundations Of Perfect Egg Quality

Regardless of how you're trying to get pregnant - whether natural or with medical assistance such as IUI or IVF - the more you strengthen nature the better.

Setting a solid foundation is critical. And it's where most people who come to me need the most help.

I remember when I was learning to play drums. I wanted to play all the fancy stuff. The crazy beats, the impressive solos. I didn't care about the basics.

For a few years I toiled away on my own and, honestly, I made some progress. By the time I enrolled in college to study Jazz Performance, I thought I really had it together.

Boy was I mistaken.

My fundamentals were - let's just say - more than slightly lacking. I was practicing for several hours every day using very poor technique.

As a result, I developed severe tendinitis in both arms and had to stop playing for a few months as a result.

After I was able to resume playing, one of my friends back in Houston who had connections with the percussion department was able to get the best teacher there - who usually only worked with the top of the top students - to accept me for lessons.

This teacher was no BS. He was completely unimpressed with me. At the first lesson he started off by asking me to just play anything I wanted, so he could get a feel for my level of skill.

5 seconds after I started, he tells me to stop.

Then he shows me the most basic, most simple exercise anyone had ever shown me. I could not believe I was finally studying with one of the world's leading teachers of jazz drums, and I'm doing what are essentially first grade lessons.

It was a slow, very precise technique, almost like "wax on, wax off" from the Karate Kid - like that.

Literally it was, "1, 2, 3, 4" super slow and with a very specific motion of the hands and stick. Over, and over, and over, and over...... and over, and over.

But, I knew this guy was the real deal, so I did as he told me. I practiced these first-grade boring exercises instead of all my complicated routines.

It forever changed my life.

I never got tendinitis again. My musical ability increased exponentially because my technique was so effortless and easy, I had a solid foundation upon which to fluidly express my ideas.

To this day, on the rare occasion when I go out and play a gig with my friends in public, people comment on how easy and relaxed I look while playing drums.

Chances are, if you're reading this book, you're like I was - way off into the complex stuff without any grounding in the most important fundamentals.

When that's the case, everything feels 10x more difficult than it is. And, in many cases by doing all the complicated diet and supplement stuff without the basics underneath, you are hurting your chances more than helping them.

Just like I was holding back my natural musical talents with my lack of fundamentals.

When I first teach my patients the Three Foundations of Perfect Egg Quality, most of them look at me with disbelief, like I have three heads.

Again, what most people are looking for is some kind of elaborate magical formula or "magic pill" and when I insist they go back to the fundamentals it's almost as if I'm insulting their intelligence.

We've become so used to pills and procedures to fix everything, we've forgotten our roots. We always want a shortcut.

The irony is that because they aren't a magic pill, they aren't a shortcut, the Three Foundations of Perfect Egg Quality are the *ultimate* shortcut. They *are* the magic pill.

When you really practice them every single day, it's like you're creating a high-speed internet connection between all your glands, organs, and tissues where before there was only a slow, unreliable, static-filled dial-up connection.

And, it's very important to remember... All these brilliant, intelligent glands, organs, cells, and tissues are more than capable of working together to create life in you.

In fact, they're already working hard every day to express nature's blueprint as best they can but, if the foundations aren't consistently in place to keep the pathways and circulation clear and open, it will be hard for them to coordinate their efforts because it will be difficult for them to communicate with each other.

Imagine you have the best team of builders ready to build your house. All the materials and the blueprints are ready to go. But, the builders can't communicate clearly because there's so much noise on the job site they can't hear each other most of the time.

They're all masters at what they do. If they were able to hear each other they'd be building the most incredible things but, because they can't, they're unable to get on the same page and start going in the same direction as a team.

That's what is happening most of the time with my patients' bodies when I first meet them. And, it's why no matter what they try in terms of supplements, herbs, diets, etc., nothing seems to work.

The master builders inside their bodies are there, ready to do their part. And even though they're getting tons of great support in the form of all those herbs and supplements and great foods…

…there's too much "static" in the system so they just can't communicate effectively. Which means the process we call "fertility" is highly inefficient and uncoordinated.

The Three Foundations Of Perfect Egg Quality solves that so that almost instantly these master builders spring into action as an unstoppable team, working together with incredible precision.

It's the ultimate shortcut. And it's insanely easy to do. It's not complicated at all and, sadly, I think this is why so few people commit to it. We're conditioned to think complicated is better.

It isn't. Especially in this case of clearing the path for nature's power to emerge in you.

Also, a lot of people are doing one or two of these, but not all three. Or, they're doing all of them but intermittently.

And that means they're just interrupting the work of those master builders - the incredibly intelligent organs and glands - that are always working to keep us alive and help us thrive.

So, the key is to do these exactly as I tell you. Don't short change yourself by doing this halfway. Realize that I have seen thousands of people just like you since 2004, and I have a massive amount of experience seeing this all day long every single day.

I know this is essential for you.

If you are already doing all these things then, great, you're ahead of the game. I still want you to follow the exact recipe I lay out for you here.

These are the soil for the seed. You can have the perfect climate and sunlight, and the right amount of water but if the soil is barren and depleted, nothing will grow.

What's the sunlight in my analogy? The mindset exercises of the first few chapters. The climate? The 7 Promises.

Later, we're going to bring it all together later with the Five Core Factors and finding your Key Signal Amplifiers which represent the water and nutrients that ensure perfect egg quality, a calm uterine environment, and stable gestation.

Also, don't make this hard. It's not difficult.

True, at first you will be required to put in some effort. That's not because these things are tiring or "hard work", it's because you're not used to doing them.

When you first tell a dog to "sit", it just looks at you having no idea what you want it to do. So, you must give it a little "push" to show it what you're asking for.

After some time, if you're patient and persistent, soon the dog will start sitting the second it knows you're telling to sit. Sometimes even before you finish saying, "Sit."

We condition our bodies to new habits the same exact way. At first, they're just not used to doing these things the way we are asking.

So, we must give them a little "push". That's the effort at the beginning.

But, after a short amount of time - like 3 to 5 days - of being consistent with our "commands" (drinking the water, going to bed at a certain time, etc.) our bodies just begin to "automatically" do them.

The ability to train our bodies to "normalize" health-promoting habits is a very powerful skill. So, use these Three Foundations as an opportunity to practice and develop this skill if you haven't already developed it.

The Three Foundations Of Perfect Egg Quality are:

1. The Embryonic Breath
2. The Perfect Hydration Plan
3. The 30 Minute Growth Hormone Accelerator

You'll find a printable "cheat sheet" to guide you through this, and the other self-care rituals in this book, in the always free **Axelrad Clinic Academy**.
Visit https://axelradclinic.com/awaken to sign up now.

PERFECT EGG QUALITY FOUNDATION ONE: The Embryonic Breath

The Embryonic Breath is a calming, gentle breathing technique that is unparalleled in how it effortlessly creates the perfect internal environment for your natural fertility to fully emerge.

Your breath is one of the most powerful tools you have for facilitating change in your physiology.

Why is this? Because it is the only "automatic" body function you can - at any time - gain conscious control of.

Why is this so important? Because your breath both reflects and controls the state of your body's stress system.

Go back to our movie theater, where I had you hooked up to all those monitors and devices. If I'm measuring respiratory rate and depth, I guarantee that during the scary movie your breathing will be more shallow and rapid, and during the love story it will be deeper and slower.

Why can I make this guarantee? *Because that's simply how your biology (and my biology, and everyone else's) works.*

When the "stress circuit" of your central nervous system is dominant, the part of your brain that controls your breathing instinctively switches you to a shallow, rapid breathing pattern. It's automatic, a biological law.

When the "relaxation circuit" of your central nervous system is dominant, the opposite happens. The part of your brain that controls breathing slows and deepens your breath.

Want more proof? OK. Think of someone sleeping. How are they breathing? Is it rapid and shallow or long and deep?

True, if someone is having a nightmare they will maybe breathe more shallow and rapid while sleeping. Otherwise, it's a nice, long, slow, deep breath.

The reason this is so important is because this is a two-way street. Meaning that not only does slow deep breathing indicate your relaxation circuit is dominant, you can MAKE your relaxation circuit dominant by intentionally slowing and deepening your breath.

We do this instinctively. Before an intense sporting event, athletes will get themselves "pumped up" by breathing more forcefully and quickly. That's because breathing this way triggers a release of cortisol and adrenaline which then triggers a heightened state of energy and alertness.

A concert pianist, on the other hand, will sit and take long, deep breaths, maybe even sigh a few times, before performing a piece in front of an audience. That's because breathing this way increases the flow of endorphins and triggers the kind of relaxed alertness that is necessary to for the calm, centered concentration it takes to perform her music at a high level.

So, by changing your breath you have powerful influence over the substances your body creates - and whether those substances are stress-positive or relaxation-positive.

Your breath is also your body's most primal rhythm, second only to your heartbeat (which is why I call it your "second heartbeat" - your sleep rhythm being the third and, of course, your actual heartbeat being the first).

And, rhythm is supremely important when it comes to creating life.

You may not realize this, but your fertility cycle is a rhythm, a wave, underneath which there are 10,000 other waves, or rhythms.

In fact, FSH and LH, along with every single other hormone in your body, are released in PULSES, not continuously. There is a rhythm to how your body secretes every single hormone in your body.

When your body wants to secrete more FSH or LH, it adjusts the rhythm. It either starts beating faster, or it beats louder, or both. And, when it wants to secrete less, it beats slower, or softer.

Your entire hormonal system is a massive symphony of rhythm, of primal drum beats. And, that symphony is set against a background of heart pulses, brain waves, breath, sleep patterns, seasonal patterns, and 1000s of other rhythms of nature.

So, by creating rhythm with your breath (and your hydration and sleep, as we'll discuss in the other two "foundations"), you're massively amplifying nature's power inside your body.

But, there's another even more cool thing to this.

When you take in deep abdominal breaths like the one I teach in The Embryonic Breath, your diaphragm expands downwards and squeezes your lower abdominal and pelvic organs.

This squeezes out old blood and with it the natural byproducts of metabolism like carbon dioxide and oxidative chemicals.

Then, when you exhale and relax the diaphragm, the downward pressure releases and a rush of fresh blood - including oxygen, nutrients, and hormones - enters.

In other words, The Embryonic Breath is like a heartbeat pumping old blood out of and fresh blood into your ovaries and uterus. It is a powerful way to maximize the circulation to your eggs and your uterine lining, so they function at the highest possible level.

Remember, I said above that blood is a LIVING tissue, a carrier of data and intelligence.

The Embryonic Breath increases the amount of life and intelligence that enters the ovarian and uterine space.

Also, want to know why I call it The Embryonic Breath?

Because if you have ever seen an embryo (which we now have the power to do thanks to the IVF process and the high-tech incubators that have been developed), you'll notice that the embryo has a subtle "pulse". The entire embryo gently pulsates.

To me this represents the *original* heartbeat of life and is essentially the embryo "breathing".

In other words that pulsing is *your* original breath because, don't forget, *you* were an embryo.

The Embryonic Breath is a way to replicate that original, rhythmic, pulsatile breathing that you had when you were an embryo. And, by doing so I truly believe that you are connecting with the deep cellular memory of how to create life.

Remember, in Chapter 3, where I reminded you about Seed Intelligence and how powerful you are? That you - as an embryo - created yourself and consciously came into this world?

The Embryonic Breath is designed to reawaken that power and conscious creative energy. And, if you do it regularly, you will find it does just that.

And, there's another bonus. It helps you achieve deep relaxation.

Patients of mine that practice this routinely report they don't get stressed as easily. They feel like things at work and home that used to bother them are no longer causing as much tension. They also tell me their sleep is more restful and it's easier to fall asleep.

How You'll Do This

1. Find a quiet place where you can sit, undisturbed, for at least 10 minutes.
2. Sit either on a cushion on the floor with your legs crossed, or on a chair. Do not lean against a wall or the back of the chair. You want to sit up in a comfortable, dignified posture.
3. You don't have to keep your spine perfectly straight, just make sure you're not slumping forward too much.
4. Close your eyes and focus all your attention on your breath.
5. Gently breathe in, letting your belly expand as you inhale.
6. Breathe out naturally, effortlessly. No push.
7. The breath should be completely silent. This is not an "ujjayi" breath as in yoga where you make a sound.
8. Count four on the inhale, four on the exhale, to make the breath perfectly even.
9. Just sit like this, breathing evenly, quietly, gently… In and out, in and out. No effort, no strain, no tension.
10. If it helps, count. I usually count backwards from 50 or 100, counting on each exhale.

And, that's it. It's that simple. There's no magic to it, but it is pure magic once you really settle into it.

Guided audio tracks for this and the other exercises in this book are waiting for you in The Axelrad Clinic Academy. It's FREE, no strings attached.

For details, visit https://axelradclinic.com/awaken.

Common Questions

What if I can't settle down and focus on the breathing?

Be patient with yourself. Depending on how wound up you are, it may take 3, 5, or even 7 ten-minute sessions to start really feeling things settle. Just commit and go all in. Trust that it's going to work.

If you give it time, I promise it will.

What if I can't stop thinking about stuff?

You don't have to stop thinking. You just have to stop letting your thoughts be your primary focus.

I have a saying for when I teach meditation: "Your heart beats, your mind thinks."

You can't stop your heartbeat, you can't stop your thoughts - as long as you're alive. So, stop trying.

Just focus on your breath, and let the thoughts be in the background. Once your thoughts are no longer "the star of the show", they'll calm down. It's all the attention you put on them that gets them excited.

So, each time you find yourself getting lost in thoughts, just come back to your breath, immediately. No hard feelings, no guilt for letting go of what you were thinking about even if it seemed important.

Your thoughts won't hold it against you, and you can always think about these things later. For now, just allow yourself to *be*.

Do I have to do this every day?

If you want it to work, yes.

And, it will work even better if you do it around the same time every day. My favorite time to do this is right before bed. It's a great way to create a little buffer between waking and sleeping, to let go of the stress of the day so I can rest peacefully.

PERFECT EGG QUALITY FOUNDATION TWO: The Perfect Hydration Plan

The Perfect Hydration Plan is a water drinking schedule that is harmonized with metabolic rhythms and is designed to:

1. Ensure continuous hydration
2. Optimize the energy available for metabolism
3. Promote ongoing gentle detoxification, and
4. Maintain clear signal pathways for your glands and organs to communicate.

Water is nothing short of a miraculous substance.

Take two of the most flammable elements in the known Universe - hydrogen and oxygen - and merge them into a substance that serves as both a coolant AND cellular fuel?

Absolute GENIUS.

It is the key to all life as we know it.

It is the basis for blood which is a liquid tissue that serves as the bridge between spirit, mind, and body.

What do I mean by "liquid tissue that serves as the bridge between spirit, mind, and body"? Simple.

When you're happy (a state of mind fueled by the spiritual qualities of hope, joy, and gratitude), your body secretes certain hormones and neurotransmitters (such as serotonin and dopamine) which are then transmitted to all your cells, glands, tissues, and organs (your body) via a special liquid flowing through an intricate network of vessels (your blood).

In fact, a single drop of your blood contains billions of bits of information about your state because the signals your body is generating in order to create that state are all contained in your blood.

People forget that follicular fluid - that amazing drop of living water that nourishes and informs the egg, the seed of life, during its growth and maturation - is derived from blood.

It is an even MORE refined signal medium. In fact, I see it as the medium for the transmission of the blueprint of creation.

That single drop of fluid that fills each follicle is a concentrated essence of who you are. Your thoughts and feelings, the foods you've eaten, both recently and over time, the relative state of vitality and self-expression of every single tissue in your body - all of these are reflected in your blood and then distilled down into a refined fluid-essence inside your follicle.

And drinking water is the most powerful way to clarify and amplify all that vital information.

Not only that, but inadequate water - what I call chronic low-grade dehydration - is one of the most effective ways to *block* that vital information from reaching your egg (not to mention one of the most stressful states for your body to deal with).

AND, water is critical for stable metabolism and healthy liver function - both of which are critical for hormonal balance and proper egg growth.

I often get blank stares from people when I tell them to ditch the flavored drinks, teas, smoothies, energy drinks, flavored "vitamin" waters, sparkling waters, and only drink good old-fashioned plain-Jane water.

Some will tell me they don't like water. Some say it'll make them have to pee too often. There's a lot of other resistance I hear.

Bottom line, I don't get anything out of you doing this or not. I'm not recommending it because it makes me feel better.

I'm recommending it because based on my clinical experience working with thousands of women who successfully had babies after years of trying, it is a powerful way to massively boost your body's ability to follow nature's life-creation blueprint to completion.

How You'll Do It

1. Get a pack of water bottles – 0.5L each bottle (or a refillable bottle of your choosing).
2. DO NOT obsess over the details on this. It's ok if the bottles are plastic. It's OK if it's not artesian water from a perfectly pristine source. You aren't going to find perfect water. If it's EASY enough then please by all means get the highest quality possible you can. But, regular bottled water will do for this. Your body can handle a few toxins, what it can't handle is dehydration.
3. Make sure it's plain water, not sparkling water. It doesn't have to be "alkaline" water either. Just plain old water will do.

The Schedule

1. Drink a bottle of water before you eat breakfast, lunch, and dinner.

2. Then, set an alarm on your phone for the following times: 10am, 2pm, 5pm, and 8pm.

3. Each time the alarm sounds, drink a full bottle of water. You can do it! Take the time you need, but you should be able to drink the whole bottle in about five minutes or less.

4. When it's time to drink the water stop everything else and just focus on drinking your water. As you do, imagine the water is carrying calming, rejuvenating energy into every cell in your body. You can imagine this as a calm, light feeling spreading through your body.

5. Don't drink any juice, flavored or caffeinated beverages during the day. (One cup of coffee in the morning is OK if you want but after a few days of adjustment along with the energizing effects of the water you're drinking, you won't need it anymore. So, feel free to stop coffee if you want after that.)

You'll find a printable "cheat sheet" to guide you through this, and the other self-care rituals in this book, in the always free **Axelrad Clinic Academy**.

Visit https://axelradclinic.com/awaken to sign up now.

Common Questions

What if I'm not thirsty?

When we're chronically dehydrated we often aren't thirsty because our bodies build a tolerance to mild dehydration. Most of my patients who start drinking water as I recommend will tell me that they start to feel very thirsty once they start my hydration plan. This thirst does subside after a few days so don't worry. So, you might have to "force it" at first, but you'll be OK after that.

Really? No smoothies?

Honestly, I think plant foods are amazing superfoods. The problem is that when fruits are liquified the sugars are released and are very rapidly absorbed into the bloodstream then converted to glucose. If you're going to do a plant-based drink, stick to green vegetables like celery, kale, and other greens and at the most add a small amount of apple or blueberries to lightly sweeten. To me, THAT'S a real smoothie. ☺

Can I drink green tea or use flavor packs for my water?

I recommend you not do this. At most, use cucumber or fresh lime or lemon and only a little bit. I just want you to drink good old-fashioned water. Sure, there are good chemicals and antioxidants in green tea and a lot of bottled water companies try to sell you flavored water with vitamins and antioxidants but for the purposes of what we're doing here, avoid these things.

Will the plastic bottles hurt me? Is it better to drink out of glass or ceramic?

Just drink the water. We're not trying to do this perfectly, we want it to be as easy and simple as possible. Often, by adding the step of having a glass or ceramic container and having to fill it from a purified source, it becomes difficult to maintain the hydration levels I'm recommending here. Trust me, you're going to be healthier and have much healthier follicles drinking 3 liters from plastic bottles than you will drinking a half or barely one liter from a glass or ceramic container.

What if I don't like water?
I don't know what to say to this other than you only *think* you don't like water. I guarantee your body LOVES water. In fact, your body craves water as much as it craves sunlight and freedom.

So, try your best to just "get over it", and get busy feeding your body an abundant quantity of the very source of life.

PERFECT EGG QUALITY FOUNDATION THREE: The 30-Minute Growth Hormone Accelerator

The 30-Minute Growth Hormone Accelerator is a pre-sleep routine that ensures deep, restful sleep which:

1. Maximizes and optimizes your adrenal circadian rhythm
2. Creates maximum resilience to physical and emotional stress
3. Calms and stabilizes immune function
4. Minimizes unnecessary inflammation, and
5. Builds an abundant supply of reserve energy.

Rest is essential for your body to replenish and regenerate. It is the foundation of tissue healing and the most powerful anti-inflammatory there is.

When you rest, your body's core temperature drops, and critical regenerative processes commence that are essential for your body's ongoing recovery from normal everyday life.

We don't think of just normal activities as stressful, but our bodies work hard just doing everyday stuff like walking, mental concentration, etc.

Sleep is nature's most powerful medicine. Period.

In fact, the *only* time your body secretes Growth Hormone - which has been shown to improve egg quality during IVF cycles in "poor responders" - is during deep, restorative REM sleep.

And this Growth Hormone is not only a massive boost for egg quality, it accelerates the repair and regeneration of microcapillaries. These are the tiny blood vessels - just big enough for a single blood cell to pass through.

These microcapillaries supply your follicles with oxygen, nutrients, hormones, and pretty much everything they need to grow and nurture a healthy egg.

Sleep is also critical for neuroendocrine balance meaning it supports healthy mood and hormonal pulses.

That's something you may not know - that hormones are pulsed. It's just like your heartbeat. As the need for a certain hormone increases, the pulse changes. High FSH is nothing more than a rapid, out of sync pulse.

So not only is sleep itself important, but your sleep rhythm is just as - if not more - important.

In fact, in my system your sleep rhythm is so important I call it your third heartbeat - the other two being your actual heartbeat and your breath.

Therefore, regulating your sleep rhythm is one of the most powerful and effective ways to bring balance to hormonal rhythms including FSH, LH, which form the basis for healthy ovulation.

Even if you're doing IVF - which circumvents your own FSH and LH - adequate sleep ensures optimal circulation and follicle growth. So, it's still a core factor.

Finally, and just as important as the anti-inflammatory, neuroendocrine balancing, growth-promoting properties of sleep is its role in stable metabolic function.

Meaning sleep is also a critical healing tool for PCOS and is key to achieving and maintaining a healthy body weight.

How You'll Do It

1. Make sure you do all your pre-sleep routine (like brushing teeth, removing make-up, getting into your sleepwear) so that you have 30 free minutes before you intend to be sleeping.
   a. Example: If you want to be asleep at 10pm (which is the time I recommend at a minimum), you need to be ready to get in bed with all pre-sleep stuff complete by 9:30pm. (FOR THE PURPOSES OF THIS WE WILL USE 10PM AS THE SLEEP TIME).
2. Get in bed at 9:30pm.
3. Make sure all electronics are turned off or in silent mode. This includes phones, tablets, e-readers, and TV.
4. Also turn off all bright overhead lighting. A reading lamp is all you'll need
5. Get some inspirational reading material. Whatever works for you. Make sure it's something that is uplifting for you.
6. Read for about 10 minutes, then close the book, turn out the lights, and lie down to sleep.

7. Begin doing your Embryonic Breath which is relaxed yet deep.

8. Start at the number 50 and count backwards from 50 to 1 – counting a number on each out-breath.

9. If you don't fall asleep after the first 50, just start back over at 50 again. Keep counting and breathing, letting all your muscles relax.

10. Within 20 minutes you will likely be asleep. If not, just stay in the dark and rest. This is the best thing you can do for your body, mind, and hormonal balance.

Common Questions

What if I have to stay up late working?

It's better to keep your bedtime the same and wake up EARLIER. Your hormonal rhythm is much less upset by waking up early than it is by going to sleep late.

Also, if you find that you are constantly behind on your work, continually staying up late, you have got to make a choice. What's more important, work and money and status, or having your baby?

Sometimes you think you want something, but how you are living says otherwise.

Also, ask yourself, "Why am I up working late, while everyone else seems to be leaving on time or working normal hours?"

Or, it may be different question, such as, "Why is the culture at my job all about working way too many hours and not having any personal time?"

Either way, stand up for yourself, and claim your space. Nobody else is going to do it for you.

What if I tend to wake up in the middle of the night?
If you wake up at night, and it seems like you are having difficulty falling back to sleep, the best thing you can do is simply stay in bed, in the dark, and rest. Don't turn on any lights, don't start looking at your phone or tablet or TV. Just rest.

If your mind is racing, using the Embryonic Breath to calm your mind and focus back on gentle, relaxed breathing.

What if it takes a while for me to fall asleep?
That's fine. Again, just stay in the dark and rest. Learn how to be still. Let your body enjoy the cool, dark, quiet space.

It is a gift.

Do Not Underestimate The Power Of This

Do not underestimate the combined power of these three rituals. It is not hyperbole to say that by doing all three of these you are exponentially increasing nature's ability to do its work in your body.

The other thing these core rituals will do is give you unbelievable psychological and emotional strength.

What I've found, over and over, is that as my patients and patients build strength, they start to find it easier and easier to know exactly what to do next. They start to tune into a deeper sense of knowing and trust in their own intuition.

Once you put these rituals into action in your life, you'll see. I promise you will NOT be disappointed.

Chapter 9 - The Sun Cycle Diet

If you're like most of the people I've worked with over the years, you've been wondering what the "best" fertility diet is.

There's a lot of information out there and a lot of possible routes to take. None of them are inherently wrong. Some are probably better than others.

But, the bottom line is, after a decade of doing this for real with literally thousands of people, I've come up with something that seems to work really, really well.

It's not really based on one diet - like Paleo or Keto or South Beach. It's a combination of all of them.

But, most importantly, it's takes biorhythms into account - in particular the 24-hour circadian rhythm.

Your body secretes cortisol, one of the most critical hormones it makes, in a 24-hour wave. First thing in the morning, your cortisol is at its peak level, and through the day it gradually declines until, at bedtime, it is at its lowest level.

Here's the thing… This cortisol wave is absolutely, inextricably, and unequivocally linked to the rising and setting of the sun.

It's inescapable and no matter what you do, no matter how much you wish it were otherwise, it can't be any different. It is simply a biological fact that cortisol levels follow the rising and setting of the sun.

169

Is it possible for this cortisol wave to shift out of rhythm a little? Yes. If you get into the habit of sleeping late or going to bed at irregular times, your cortisol wave will definitely shift.

That's because your body loves you so much, it will always try to adapt to what you throw at it.

But, just because your body *can* do it, doesn't mean it's good for you.

Bottom line is there's no such thing as a nocturnal human - a "night owl" as we often say when speaking of someone who likes to stay up late at night or function on minimum hours of sleep.

(This may seem like a digression because, after all, I'm supposed to be telling you about a diet. And, I'm going to get to that but first I want to make sure you know how important it is for you to harmonize EVERYTHING with this 24-hour rhythm.)

It is absolutely not optional to sync up with the natural day-night cycle if you want to give yourself the absolute best chance to get pregnant. I don't care whether you're overweight or underweight, doing IVF or trying on your own, 25 or 45 years of age... This 24-hour cortisol circadian rhythm is the key to your salvation. Literally.

So, you've already learned The Three Foundations which, when applied, will sync your sleep, hydration, and breathing so they support and strengthen this vital rhythm.

Now, you're going to learn what I call The Sun Cycle Diet.

What It Is

This is more than just a "what to eat, what not to eat" thing. Yes, there are foods you want to avoid as much as possible, and foods you want to emphasize.

We'll get to that soon.

But, the real magic of this diet is the WHEN. It's the timing of your meals, and what those meals are composed of at those specific times.

In short, this diet harnesses your body's innate metabolic rhythm to maximize inner strength and minimize things that disrupt your fertility cycle.

It's very easy to do, but it may represent a change for you. That's because most of us (in the West, anyway) were raised on small breakfasts and big dinners. We were indoctrinated into the false belief that fat is harmful, that fruit is always healthy, and that we need a balance between all the five "food groups" which, we're told, are meat, dairy, grains, vegetables, and fruits.

Here's the thing - grains are not essential. Fruits are not essential. Vegetables are not essential. Dairy is not essential.

You can live a very healthy, long, prosperous life without ANY of those foods.

True, plants are amazing foods rich in nutrients and - obviously - I'm not saying you shouldn't eat them. I'm just saying they're not *essential*.

There are only three *essential* foods - protein, fat, and water.

You may be shaking your head right now thinking I'm out of my mind. And, I don't blame you. Since the beginning you've been indoctrinated into the food group myth.

But I promise, it is a fact that:

1. Animal protein contains all essential amino acids to build every single type of cell, tissue, or substance your body needs, along with every vitamin and mineral you need to thrive, and
2. Animal fat, which is nothing more than a huge, extremely complicated mass of sugar molecules, contains all the glucose you need to generate more than enough cellular energy.

You literally don't need anything else than this. Not that I'm going to tell you NOT to eat anything else... so don't jump ahead of me. ;-)

I know this is potentially a controversial view. And, I understand some people are uncomfortable with it because, after all, it flies in the face of the deep nutritional dogma we've all grown up with.

But, all I can say is that over and over and over I've seen it work. I've seen people who'd been trying for years, or who'd suffered through multiple failed IVFs, adopt the Sun Cycle Diet and it was after that they got to a place where they produced an egg healthy enough to become a baby - and a body strong enough to carry it.

How You'll Do This

The diet is incredibly simple. Again, *do not make it complicated.* Yes, it is probably a change for you, but I know you can do it.

And, like everything else in this book, I am 100% confident that once you start it you'll never look back. It will change your life and at the same time massively increase nature's ability to work through you and complete its life-creation blueprint.

You'll find a printable "cheat sheet" to guide you through this, and the other self-care rituals in this book, in the always free **Axelrad Clinic Academy**.
Visit https://axelradclinic.com/awaken to sign up now.

Step 1 – Eat a large, protein-dense breakfast, as close to zero carbs as possible.

In the morning, as the sun is rising, your metabolism is also "rising". It is in a fragile state, like a fire that has just been started from embers. You must protect it and nurture it so that it can grow into a full, self-sustaining fire. If you overload it or don't give it enough fuel, either way you damage it.

Imagine a pond at dawn that is completely still, not a single wave, like glass. That's your metabolism before your first meal.

If you eat sugar, carbs, or grains and your blood sugar spikes - and along with it your insulin - it is like throwing a huge rock into the pond and creating massive waves that will likely take all day to settle back down.

Literally that one meal will set the table for your entire day from a metabolic standpoint.

So, the key for the morning meal is *simplicity*.

173

Example: Eggs and turkey bacon. The only carb that is OK here is a small amount of oatmeal if you really want it. Also, as per the Perfect Hydration Plan, drink only water. No juice.

Step 2 – Eat a diverse, low-carb, satisfying lunch, with the size dictated by your appetite.

At noon, your metabolism, like the sun, is at its zenith. The fire is burning at full heat. Especially if you've set the table properly with the right kind of zero-sugar morning meal and plenty of water.

At this time, you can eat a more varied - and larger - meal. That's because the fire is ready to consume whatever you put into it.

But, it's still important to exercise restraint and make sure you don't spike your insulin by eating sugars and starches in large quantities. I prefer you don't eat them at all, but during lunch a little rice or quinoa or wheat-free pasta is fine. Key word - a *little*.

Still, the key for the mid-day meal is *variety*.

Example: Hamburger patty with lettuce, tomato, avocado.

Step 3 – Eat a healthy snack around 3 hours after lunch.

Mid-afternoon your metabolic fire, like the sun, is still burning hot so it's a good time to feed your body a little extra nutrition heading into the evening.

Plus, as you see below in step 4, dinner isn't going to be so big, so this is a good time to "stock up", so to speak.

Example: Celery with almond butter (it's better than you think).

174

Step 4 – Eat a small, simple, protein-dense dinner that has plenty of healthy fats

In the evening, your metabolism is waning, like the setting sun. It is winding down to prepare for rest and rejuvenation during sleep.

Think of a campfire, after it has burned all day and is down to the embers. The last thing you want to do is throw a bunch of wood on it at this point. It will smother the coals and you end up with no fire and bunch of half-burned wood.

Remember, while you sleep, your metabolism slows down dramatically, and your body temperature drops 1 - 2 degrees lower than normal. If you eat a large meal now, your body will be overwhelmed, and your metabolism will not be able to handle it appropriately.

So, at this point, you want your meal to be small and - again - simple.

Therefore, the key to the evening meal is *restraint*. You must eat small - even just a snack-sized portion, and keep it very, very simple.

Example: Chicken breast with broccoli or Beef with Brussel sprouts or Salmon with asparagus.

Some Important Keys

1. Be realistic. There is no special prize for being perfect. You can still have fun.
2. This way of eating should be thought of as a "weekday diet". Do not be so rigid that you always eat this way, at the expense of enjoying a weekly night out with friends and family, etc.
3. The key is that you don't deviate too far from the plan, and not for too long. Pick and choose your days off and get back on the plan as soon as possible.

4. For this reason, I recommend you be VERY STRICT for the first 2 weeks. This "initiation period" will help you establish the pattern more strongly. Then, when you do go out for that late-night meal with friends on a Friday night, it will be easy to stay locked in on Saturday night.

Basic Food Lists

Here are some basic "do's and don'ts" as far as foods to focus on and foods to steer away from. This is intentionally simple because - at the end of the day - this is supposed to be easy for you.

Food is an insanely complex area - there are so many different types of foods, so many different combinations and recipes... It is - in my opinion - one of the easiest places to overcomplicate and very quickly get lost.

So, keep this as simple as possible and follow this basic plan:

Anytime, anywhere:
- Beef
- Chicken
- Fish (deep ocean only)
- Lean pork
- Eggs
- Other free-range meats such as deer, buffalo, etc. if that's your thing.

Eat as much as you want, within reason:
- Leafy greens
- Cruciferous veggies like broccoli, cauliflower
- Gourds - this includes squash, zucchini, cucumber
- Nuts

Eat in extreme moderation:
- Root vegetables - carrots, potatoes (yes, even sweet potatoes) - these tend to have more sugar and starches.
- Fruit - again, more sugar than you think. Stick to apples, tart berries and avoid super-sweet fruits like pineapple, grapes.
- Brown rice, quinoa.

Eat almost never:
- White rice.
- Legumes - this includes soy, peanuts, most beans.

Eliminate completely if possible:
- Wheat flour and anything made with it like bread, cookies, cake, pasta
- Animal dairy - especially milk
- Any heavily processed foods like cured meats, dried fruits

Common Questions

Why no wheat flour?

First thing - and this is very important - by telling you not to eat wheat flour *I am not saying "gluten-free"*.

I'm simply saying don't eat wheat flour.

There are tons of "gluten-free" products out there that still contain large quantities of refined wheat flour. And, it's the refined part, along with the wheat part, that is the problem.

The wheat that is available for consumption today is not the same wheat our ancestors ate. It is highly genetically modified and, in my opinion, extremely harmful if consumed regularly over a long period of time.

I don't take lightly what I just said, because I'm not an alarmist, nor am I a conspiracy theorist.

But I truly believe that the wheat put out on the market today is simply not fit for human consumption and should be avoided if possible.

Of course, if you want to eat a little bit on occasion, it's not going to kill you and it won't block your fertility. Your body is stronger than that.

But, avoid it for a few days and you'll understand what I mean. You'll feel it. Trust me.

Also, wheat flour is extremely reactive with your body's insulin/metabolic axis. In fact, it can be worse than refined sugar in many respects.

Again, insulin is the biggest disrupter of hormonal communications. It is literally like a "pause button" on hormonal rhythm. Everything stops when your insulin spikes.

In fact, avoiding wheat flour and moderating fruit consumption eliminates 80-90% of the sugar from your diet, pretty much instantly. So, it's the proverbial "low-hanging fruit" of sugar elimination and insulin stabilization.

Why no dairy?

Pretty simple here. There is no animal in nature that consumes mother's milk after infancy. Not one.

Even though that's pretty much all you need to know, I'll explain further because I know there is a massive amount of dogma around dairy being good for you, being necessary for healthy bones and teeth, and other things that simply aren't true.

First, store-bought milk - whether "organic" or not, or whether from grass-fed or corn-fed, or hormone & antibiotic-free animals - is highly processed.

Pasteurization and homogenization completely change the structure of the milk and, in my opinion, makes it unnatural to consume.

Secondly, milk is a growth-promoting substance, created by nature to support rapid growth and development of the immune system in infants.

Therefore, it is a highly reactive substance in terms of hormones AND immune function and I simply do not feel it is beneficial for any adult to consume outside of a situation where there is literally nothing else to eat.

And that's probably how people started drinking milk after infancy, anyway.

It was likely out of pure necessity - like a winter after a bad harvest. In that situation it provided much needed and powerful nourishment to stay alive. Plus, we're talking about milk straight from the source, unprocessed, and consumed immediately.

Another final word about dairy. And, that word is *lactose*.

Lactose is… sugar. And sugar, again, triggers insulin secretion. Especially when that sugar is unaccompanied by fiber. Last time I checked, milk contains no fiber.

What about my smoothies?

Bottom line, smoothies in my opinion are not ideal.

Yes, it's true, there's a huge industry around selling you the idea that smoothies are super-healthy - then selling you the supplies and the equipment to make them.

But, in the end, I think they should be consumed rarely if at all and should NOT be used to substitute for eating nourishing, high-protein foods for breakfast.

Additionally, most people incorrectly assume that a couple of apples or grapes to sweeten a smoothie is no big deal.

I disagree. The sugar released when these fruits are liquified becomes at least 2-3x more potent and the resulting insulin spike is a major hormonal disruptor.

Stick to food - real food - whenever possible.

If I'm not drinking milk, where will I get my calcium?

Milk, contrary to the brilliant marketing by the industry that produces it, is not necessary for healthy bones and teeth in adults.

Eating leafy greens along with animal protein is more than enough to cover your calcium needs. You simply don't need the high levels of calcium in fortified dairy milk and - in fact - it is now proven that cardiovascular disease, dementia, and many other "diseases of aging" are, in fact, related in large part to calcium deposits forming in vital tissues including organs and blood vessels.

In other words, we are literally becoming "calcified" by our overzealous dairy consumption.

But what if I don't have time for breakfast?

This is something I'm not able to understand, honestly. As with all things, you either choose to make the time, or you don't.

Breakfast is absolutely the most critical meal of the day. That's because your body is in a fasting state in the morning. You haven't eaten in several hours and your cortisol system and adrenal glands are in desperate need of help.

Not eating breakfast is absolutely one of the most - if not *the* most - self-destructive dietary habits when it comes to maintaining hormonal rhythms and taking proper care of your body. Maybe only second to chronic low-grade dehydration from not drinking enough water.

So, bottom line is, *make the time*. Do what you must do. I wish I had a way around this for you, but there simply isn't one.

Like I said at the very beginning of the book, you can't bribe nature, you can't bargain with nature. She simply does not care about your busy schedule. She wants you to feed your body and she's not going to compromise on that.

You can do this. I promise.

The Sun Cycle Diet is insanely simple. It just boils down to:
1. No wheat flour or animal dairy.
2. Lots of green veggies and animal protein.
3. Minimal grains and legumes.
4. Sensible meal times and sizes that follow natural metabolic rhythms.

Keep it simple and do it. I guarantee you'll feel amazing and you'll never want to go back to whatever you were doing before.

Chapter 10 - The Truth About Exercise & Fertility - It's Probably Not What You Think

(IMPORTANT: It can be dangerous to do certain exercises during the stimulation phase of an IVF cycle, and when taking certain medications. If you are doing or planning an IVF cycle, follow the advice and instructions of your doctor to the letter.)

In this chapter I'm going to teach you a very basic yet very powerful exercise routine that, in my experience, is very, very helpful to support strength, resilience, and - most importantly - hormonal clarity.

It's a very moderate, easy, and brief routine designed to be done daily for about 10-15 minutes in the morning. This should make it easy for anyone to incorporate into daily life.

This exercise routine gently stretches and strengthens, requires no equipment, no special training or trips to the gym. It is, in short, designed to guarantee success because there is simply no way anyone can make the excuse that it's too difficult, too time consuming, too expensive, or too tiring.

I'll explain the details on the method at the end of this chapter. But first, I want to make sure I clear some things up.

The Controversy About Exercise And Fertility

Exercise is - bar none - probably the most "controversial" area within the realm of fertility medicine. And, I'm not going to shy away from it.

You'll hear "you shouldn't exercise too much if you're trying to get pregnant" and, in general, I do believe excessive exercise can have negative effects on fertility.

The problem is… what do we mean by "excessive"?

In my opinion - as long as you're not a hardcore endurance athlete - if you're already in great shape you should *not* stop exercising.

In fact, I think being in shape helps you a lot, in many ways.

My sister was an avid runner for years and ran 6 miles every morning. She didn't have any issues getting pregnant the first time in her mid-thirties and then again the third time in her late-thirties. She even had to be told by her doctor to stop running at 16 weeks after she had some cramps after one of her runs.

However, the reason her running didn't impact her fertility like it might for someone else is simply this: She was in that kind of shape for a long, long time and - for her - that 6-mile run was EASY. (I know this because once - emphasis here on ONCE - I went on a run with her and while I was desperately sucking wind she was talking to me as if nothing was happening for the entire six miles).

The first thing I want to say before I get into the details of how I teach my patients to exercise is this - the way most people exercise in Western cultures today is either one extreme or the other. It's either unnecessarily extreme and taxing OR, conversely, woefully inadequate.

Both situations are just as harmful and cause the exact same result - depleted energy reserves, chronic systemic inflammation, metabolic shifts that do not favor fertility, and long-term tissue degeneration.

The Unnecessary Toll Of Excessive Exercise

What I'm referring to here is the obsession with endurance, speed, chiseled physiques, and breaking through physical limits. Ironmans, CrossFit, hardcore spinning, marathons, triathlons…

It's important to recognize that while our bodies were designed to move, stretch, and reach, they were not designed for this kind of brutal punishment.

Let's be clear. I'm not *criticizing* people who do this kind of extreme athletic training.

Honestly, I admire people who want to challenge themselves and reach for their goals and who have the discipline and willpower to do things like run 26.2 miles or spend 2 hours in a gym flipping truck tires and leaping onto tall boxes and climbing rock walls.

But, let's be real. All extreme athletes end up with physical ailments. Joint problems, muscle and tendon and ligament tears… It's always a "no-pain, no-gain" proposition.

The reason these injuries start to occur sooner or later is because the body of an extreme athlete is not given enough recovery time - ever. And, that leads to chronic, ongoing degenerative changes that eventually end up in tissue breakdown.

Our bodies are incredibly intelligent. If we don't rest, they'll do everything they can to go along with the demands but, at some point, they will force us to give them time to heal.

It's either your choice or your body's choice. If it's your body's choice, we call that "injury".

185

I think it's obvious where I'm going with this.

If you are trying to get pregnant and you are training at a serious athletic level, and you're NOT getting pregnant, then it's very likely related to the demands you're putting on your physical body and, specifically, the inflammation you're generating.

Inflammation is a natural stage in the healing process and isn't inherently bad. It only becomes "bad" when it becomes chronic, as your body is never allowed the space to complete the healing cycle.

Now, I can't tell you why some people run marathons and still get pregnant without much of a problem, and others do not.

All I know is, if you're an extreme exerciser and you're reading this book, you need to dial it back. It's time.

I believe there is always a compulsion of some type that drives people to exercise excessively (and, yes, I believe marathons and severe spinning classes and a lot of the high-intensity workout stuff out there is excessive). Roughly half the time it's appearance-driven, half the time it's status driven.

In other words, if you feel compelled to push your athletic limits its either because you derive a large part of your self-esteem based on a certain look or belonging to a certain tribe of "high-performers".

We all must make sacrifices to get what we want sometimes. I get how important it might be for you to keep exercising at the level you are now. And, I get that you obviously know how to sacrifice because you are putting in some serious hours and effort into reaching the level you are at.

But, you're going to have to make a choice. What's more important? Having that "beach body" and being part of the "hardcore athlete set", or being a mother?

Because, it's probably going to come down to choosing one or the other.

It's not a "exercise" or "no exercise" situation, either. It doesn't have to be black-or-white. A lot of my highly athletic patients are very "Type-A" personalities who tend to paint everything in terms of "you win, or you lose". No middle ground, no compromise.

In this case, the art of compromise will serve you very, very well.

Dialing back your exercise for now, so that you can allow your body's energy reserves to replenish, your inflammatory system to recover, your metabolism to settle, your hormonal system to reset, is not a death-knell for your lifetime fitness goals.

You getting pregnant and having a child is not going to erase your motivation or your discipline to get back to doing what you love with exercise and fitness.

But, you're going to have to let go of some control of your body if you want to get pregnant. You're going to have to understand that another being is going to attach to you and your body is going to have to undergo changes in order to bring that being into the world.

And, you are not going to be able to dictate the exact nature of those changes, as you are doing now with your exercise habits.

You must step back and let nature take over. That means you might gain a few more pounds than you'd like because, well, nature KNOWS you need those fat cells to generate the estrogen necessary to feed that egg and then build and sustain the uterine lining through the first trimester.

And, this is often the hardest part for my athletic patients - surrendering control. And, you might as well start learning it now because - trust me - once your baby is here you're going to have to surrender a LOT more.

So, use this shift in exercise habits as "practice" for the next stage of your life, which is motherhood. If it's truly important to you, you'll be willing to make this sacrifice. It's that simple.

The Hidden Toll Of Insufficient Exercise Levels

Your body was designed to move - you created it that way so you could explore the world and interact with life. You were not meant to sit for several hours a day. And, doing so is just as - if not more - stressful than running a marathon.

Sedentary life depletes your energy reserves and leads to chronic inflammation just as much as excessive exercise. And the metabolic effects are a complete disaster.

Combine all of this with the massive stress sedentary life puts on your circulatory system, and you have a recipe for a total blockage of nature's life-creation blueprint.

Now, here's the key. If you're a sedentary person, you don't have to become a world-class athlete in order to provide powerful support to your body's ability to get pregnant.

That's because - as I've stated over and over - your body is incredibly resilient and intelligent and as soon as you start giving it the support it needs, it begins to heal immediately.

Not tomorrow, not in a few days or weeks or months. *Right now.*

But you must commit to it and do it every single day. Or it's not going to work very well if at all.

Why every day?

Because if you've been more-or-less sedentary for a long time, your body's hormonal and metabolic rhythm is shifted. It's essentially adapted to your lack of movement and that lower-fertility shift is your new "default".

Once your body finds a default, it wants to stay there, even if it's not the most "healthy" default. It's just the way our bodies (and minds, actually) work. They learn, they adapt, they change, and they develop habits.

So, shifting your body into a more living, productive, hormonally clear state is going to take a little bit of time and effort, but not as much time and effort as you think.

The problem when we've become sedentary is we've reached a state of inertia, and the hardest part is simply overcoming that inertia by getting started.

Also, I want to make clear that "incidental exercise" doesn't count for the purposes of what I'm teaching you here.

"Incidental exercise" means exercise that occurs as part of your daily routine.

For example, a lot of my sedentary patients will ask me if the half-mile total walk from their car to their desk counts, or if they are getting their 10,000 steps as part of their daily work routine counts as enough exercise for what I'm talking about here.

Simple answer: No, it doesn't.

At least not for the purposes of you shifting out of where you are to a place where your body will create life.

To get a different result, you're simply going to have to do different things than you're doing now.

Instead, we're going to focus on some "Sustained Intentional Movement", where you are moving your body for a sustained period with an intention to exercise.

It takes a very small amount of time - just 10-15 minutes a day, in fact - but you must focus, and keep at it. And, you must do it every single day. I'll get to that in a second, but first...

A Word About Body Image

For many, exercise is tied up in body image. And, this gets into some very, very deep psychology.

The bottom line is if you practice the self-directed loving-kindness I talk about earlier in the book, and you really, really commit to that, your body-image issues will start to dissolve on their own.

That's because body-image issues are always based in self-directed shame, fear, judgment, guilt, or anger.

So, don't JUST do this exercise thing, don't JUST do the diet thing. That might be what you've been doing up to this point - trying to manipulate your body into becoming "fertile" again without changing your emotional or psychological state.

You have got to get your mindset straightened out if you want to have the best chance for this to work. There's simply no way around it. So, keep doing the mindset rituals as you incorporate this simple exercise routine into your daily life.

If you find you're getting really, anxious about changing your exercise routine - especially if you are more of an obsessive exerciser - then you are pushing against some of these challenging emotions.

Put in a little extra time practicing self-directed loving-kindness and see if it helps you calm down. If not, then I strongly suggest you speak with a therapist that specializes in this area, to uncover and release whatever deep-seated emotional patterns are holding you back.

What This Is

This is a set of four simple exercises that stretch, strengthen, and loosen your body. They are designed to help you relax and focus while at the same time providing powerful shifts in circulation and metabolism.

They are not difficult at all. But don't let the ease and simplicity fool you. They are very powerful and precise and have powerful and positive effects on your entire body and, specifically, the clarity and power of your endocrine system.

The simplicity is on purpose, so you can learn them quickly. The ease is also on purpose, so you can do them every day and your body can fully recover every day.

The goal with these exercises is to awaken, circulate, and consolidate your body's energy and promote a state of open circulation, natural relaxation, mental clarity, and core strength.

The goal is not weight loss or extreme athletic ability. However, if you ARE overweight, and you combine this with the Sun Cycle Diet, I guarantee you will start to lose weight and feel a TON more energy as well.

If you are more athletic, you will not lose muscle tone or gain weight. However, you will not maintain "marathon-level" endurance. Which, honestly, is a GOOD thing at this stage of your life, if you're truly wanting to get pregnant and have a baby.

How You'll Do This

As I said, there are four exercises you'll do, and I'll describe them in detail below. They are derived from Yoga, Qigong, and Isometrics. You don't need any special equipment and this whole routine should take no more than 15 minutes.

Do your best to do this entire routine every single day, upon arising, before your shower. The reason I want you to do it in the morning is, again, your cortisol circadian rhythm is at its peak. You have the energy and the focus to do it.

If you are not a "morning person", this routine will help you become one by helping shift you back into sync (along with the Three Foundations). You'll start waking up with energy and feeling good in the mornings and that will be a sign you are making HUGE progress.

The four exercises are, in order:
1. Connecting Heaven And Earth
2. Swimming Dragon

3. Pushing Mountain
4. Concentrating The Heavenly Pearl

(There are video demonstrations of all these exercises in our free patient portal - which you have lifetime access to as a reader of this book. Just visit https://axelradclinic.com/awaken to sign up.)

General guidelines:

- MOVE SLOWLY. None of these are fast exercises.
- Do these every day. Make the commitment and stay steady.
- Repeat each exercise 5 times to start, eventually increasing to 10-15 reps. If you're already in pretty good shape, feel free to start at 10 reps.

General warnings:

- **If you are injecting medication to hyper stimulate your ovaries (as is often done during IUI and IVF cycles), do not do these exercises. Follow your doctor's instructions.**
- Once you are pregnant, you can continue all exercises except "Concentrating The Heavenly Pearl". Just make sure you are NOT STRAINING.
- If you have pain, dizziness, or shortness of breath, stop and lie down immediately.
- If you have diagnosed spinal, joint, or cardiovascular issues (such as hypertension, herniated discs, knee problems, etc.), please consult your doctor before starting these exercises.

Exercise One: Connecting Heaven And Earth

This exercise gently opens and stretches your spine, which is the central channel of the network of nerves that controls and regulates endocrine and circulatory function. It is also very relaxing and helps discharge stress.

193

1. Start with your feet shoulder width apart, arms relaxed at your sides, knees unlocked and slightly bent.

2. As you inhale into your belly, turn your palms up and, as you lean back just slightly arching your spine, lift your arms out to your sides, shoulders relaxed, in a sweeping motion until your hands are over your head, palms facing each other, about shoulder width apart.

3. Now exhale and bring your arms down in front of you, palms facing each other, as you bend forward, allowing your spine to curl and your knees to bend, until your belly is resting on your thighs and your hands are resting on the floor.

4. Stay in this forward bend position and relax your upper body completely. Your neck, your shoulders, your arms are completely relaxed and suspended from your waist. Your spine should be relaxed in a curve, not straight.

5. Take a couple of breaths in this position.

6. Then, as you inhale, tuck your tailbone under and roll your spine up from the bottom to the top, slowly and gently. Keep your shoulders and arms completely relaxed at your sides as you come up to a standing position.

7. Once you are upright, exhale and gently sink down, letting your knees bend just slightly.

8. Repeat steps 2-7. Start with 5 reps daily and gradually work your way up to 15-20.

Tips for doing this exercise:

- Don't scrunch your shoulders. Let your shoulders stay completely relaxed as your arms move outward and upward. An easy way to do this is to imagine your wrists are attached to strings in the ceiling and are being pulled upwards, so the movement is initiated from the wrist, not the shoulder.

- Do not come up from the forward bend with your spine straight. Doing so puts a tremendous amount of pressure on

194

your lumbo-sacral joint and could cause injury. Instead, visualize your vertebrae stacking themselves one on top of the other starting at the bottom up to the top.

Safety tips:

- **DO NOT, under ANY circumstances, do this exercise while stimming during an IVF cycle. Serious injury may result.**
- Be careful if you have a history of lower back injuries such as herniated discs. Go slow and stop immediately if you experience back pain.
- If you have high or low blood pressure as you may get dizzy going up and down. If you experience dizziness, stop and lie down on the floor face up for a few minutes until you feel better, then slowly get up.

Exercise Two: Swimming Dragon

This exercise stretches the tendons and ligaments along the spine with gentle twisting. It also gives a gentle (and completely safe) squeeze to the liver, gut, and pelvic organs.

1. At the end of the Connecting Heaven And Earth exercise, immediately inhale and bring your arms out to your sides until your hands are at shoulder level, in a "T" position, neck and shoulders relaxed.
2. Now exhale and gently twist to the left - from the waist - as you gently allow your arms to wrap around your torso.
3. Your left hand will end up behind your back, pressed up against your lumbar area, palm facing out.
4. Your right hand will end up palm down on your left shoulder.
5. Look as far over your left shoulder as possible, without straining your neck.

6. Now inhale and twist back to front, gently and gracefully moving your arms back to the "T" position.
7. Exhale and repeat the twist to the right, with the right hand moving to the lumbar area, palm up, and the left hand moving to the right shoulder.
8. Look over your right shoulder as far as you can without forcing it or straining.
9. Inhale and come back to the starting "T" position.
10. Repeat steps 2-9. Start with 5 reps daily and gradually work your way up to 15-20.

Tips for doing this exercise:

- Again, don't scrunch your shoulders. Let your shoulders stay completely relaxed as your arms move into the "T" position. An easy way to do this is to imagine your wrists are attached to strings in the ceiling and are being outwards, so the movement is initiated from the wrist, not the shoulder.
- Do not force the twist. Let it be gentle and natural.
- Initiate the twist from the WAIST, not the upper back.
- Be graceful and fluid in your movements and don't stop - once you reach the full twist immediately start inhaling and moving back to center.

Safety tips:

- **DO NOT, under ANY circumstances, do this exercise while stimming during an IVF cycle. Serious injury may result.**
- Be careful if you have a history of lower back injuries such as herniated discs. Go slow and if you experience pain stop.

Exercise Three: Pushing Mountain

This exercise works the largest muscles in your body to powerfully ramp up oxygenation of the blood. Also, strengthening and working the legs is a powerful way to increase adrenal tone and help set a strong foundation for your body's hormonal cycles.

1. Stand with your feet slightly wider than shoulder width apart, knees unlocked and slightly bent, arms relaxed at your sides, toes pointing forward.
2. Inhale and bring your hands up along the front of your body - as if you are painting the front of your torso and your hands are the brushes - until your hands are at chest level.
3. Exhale and slowly bend your knees and drop your butt as if you're going to sit on a chair, as you press your hands forward as if gently pushing against a big mountain.
4. Continue the exhale until your arms are fully extended in front of you, palms pushing away, and you are squatting down as far as you can *comfortably* go.
   a. Important note here: Use your arms as a counterbalance and push your tailbone BACK into your squat. Your weight should be on your heels, not the balls of your feet. Your knees should not move forward at all, and they should stay behind your toes. See the picture to be sure you're doing it right, as this can cause ligament injury in your knees if done improperly.
5. Now inhale and come out of your squat to a standing position as you simultaneously pull your arms back in towards you - keeping your palms facing down and bending at the elbows.
6. Once you are standing, exhale and allow your hands to sink down to your sides, arms and shoulders relaxed.
7. Repeat steps 2-6. Start with 5 reps daily and gradually work your way up to 15-20.

197

Tips for doing this exercise

- Again, don't scrunch your shoulders. Let your shoulders stay completely relaxed as your hands move up along the front of your torso. An easy way to do this is to imagine your wrists are attached to strings in the ceiling and are being outwards, so the movement is initiated from the wrist, not the shoulder.
- Be graceful and fluid in your movements and don't stop - once you reach your full squat immediately begin the inhale and come up to standing again, exhale and drop the arms, then immediately inhale your hands up the front of your body and begin the process again.

Safety tips:

- **DO NOT, under ANY circumstances, do this exercise while stimming during an IVF cycle. Serious injury may result.**
- Make sure as you "push against the mountain" you do so gently. Push too hard and you can strain ligaments and tendons in your shoulders.
- Do not let your knees push forward over your toes. This is very important as it can cause ligament damage. Just squat as much as you comfortably can and, over time, you'll stretch out more to where you can squat further without hurting yourself.

Exercise Four: Concentrating The Heavenly Pearl

This is essentially an abdominal crunch but done slowly and with intention. It gently and powerfully strengthens your core and pushes fresh blood into your pelvic organs including uterus and ovaries.

Contrary to what many believe, this is very beneficial for your fertility, especially if you tend to have a sedentary lifestyle.

Practice on a soft surface or use a soft mat. Do not do this on tile or any type of hard floor without protection.

1. Lie on your back, knees bent and thighs gently touching, soles of feet flat on the floor, hands cradling your head at the base of the skull with your elbows pointing straight up towards the ceiling.
2. Inhale gently but deeply so your belly rises.
3. As you exhale, gently squeeze your abdominal muscles to bring your elbows and knees towards each other. Your spine will curve as you do this. Try not to move your legs or arms. Let your abdominal muscles do all the work.
4. When the exhale is complete, slowly relax your abdominal muscles as you inhale.
5. As soon as your back is flat on the floor, begin your next exhale and again bring your knees and elbows towards each other using your abdominal muscles only.
6. Repeat steps 2-5. Start with 5 reps daily and gradually work your way up to 15-20.

Tips for this exercise

- Make sure all the movement of the elbows and knees towards each other is a result of you collapsing your core, not moving the legs or arms.
- If there is any pain - especially in the back or belly - stop immediately.

Safety tips:

- *DO NOT, under ANY circumstances, do this exercise while stimming during an IVF cycle. Serious injury may result.*

Important Rules To Follow

Do these daily

The key to this working is to do it *daily*. Even if you only do 5 of each, do them *daily*.

If you miss a day, just get back on track the next. Also, if you do happen to forget or just can't get them in one morning, feel free to do them later in the day that day.

Do them first thing in the morning

But, it is important to do these at the prescribed time which is first thing in the morning after you use the restroom and before you shower.

Be gentle and move slowly

These are not meant to be fast or intense. Be gentle, move slowly, take your time. Don't rush and don't try to break any records.

Part Three
Amplifying The Signal With Targeted Supplements

"I have just three things to teach: simplicity, patience, compassion.
These three are your greatest treasures."
- Lao Tzu

Chapter 11 - The Five Core Factors And Discovering Your Key Supplements

I'm going to get into some stuff here that's a little more complicated than what we have been discussing up to this point.

So, it's a good time for me to remind you of one of the core principles:

Knowledge is not power. Power is power.

You don't have to know *how* any of this works for it to work – that's because getting pregnant has nothing to do with knowing the mechanics.   At   all.

When you get into your car to drive to work, you sit behind the wheel, start the car, and start driving. The car is doing thousands of things from the second you start it until you reach your destination.

If you sat there the entire time you were driving it thinking about all the chemical reactions, gears, pressure changes, torque, electrical current modulation, and all the other things the car was doing, there's simply no way you could even make it to your destination.

You'd be completely overwhelmed. There's no way you could just focus on DRIVING THE CAR.

Your body is the same way except that - instead of thousands - there are billions upon billions of things going on outside of your conscious awareness and control. And, the parts you do control are extremely limited.

What we want to do is let go of trying to be in control of EVERYTHING and focus on what I call "The ABC Principle" which pretty much sums up the ONLY things you have any real control over.

They are, in order, your:
1. Attitude
2. Breathing
3. Choices

First, you choose the attitude with which you approach life - including its challenges, problems, victories, and defeats.

Next, you choose how you are breathing at any given moment. As we uncovered above with Embryonic Breath, when you slow and calm your breathing you create a calm, relaxed state inside your body as well.

And, finally, you choose what you're doing and what you're focusing on. What will you eat? What time will you go to sleep? How will you react to something someone says? What are your priorities?

Focus on the ABC's, and life becomes very, very simple.

Up until now, I've taught you some very important mindset, diet, and movement techniques that form the daily foundation of the Awakening The Seed process.

In fact, if you *only* do these things, and do them with focus and commitment, you've already at least doubled or tripled your fertility.

All these techniques are designed to help you tap into the vast amount of power you already embody – the very power that created all life.

Yes, you are an embodiment of that. Don't ever forget it.

I've also helped you see that much, if not all, of what you believed about your ability to get pregnant is nothing more than elaborate mythology – stories that may be true for others but certainly aren't true in the general sense. And, that you can let go of those myths, so you don't continue to limit your story going forward.

We also talked about the Six Laws Of Seed Intelligence, which help you tap into your innate power and intuition.

And, we've outlined the Seven Core Promises which are a list of commitments you make to yourself – to hold yourself accountable so that you stay on track.

These laws and promises are like the bedrock upon which this entire system operates. Without them you're just doing the same thing you were doing before – trying this, trying that, going in circles, and getting frustrated, anxious, and overwhelmed.

We've also talked about The Sun Cycle Diet, a way of eating that ensures your body is always nourished in a way that falls in line with natural metabolic rhythms. Eating in this way takes all the stress off your metabolic system and creates a maximal healing opportunity for all your cells, glands, and organs.

Now it's time to discuss what I call…

The Five Core Factors

This is where we start to look at specific supplements you can take to further "take it up a notch" in helping your Seed Intelligence to emerge and break through.

204

Remember, nature only needs a tiny opening to break through. It doesn't need perfection. It only needs "good enough".

You don't have to do this perfectly and certainly you don't have to take every possible supplement that might help.

In fact, you don't even have to do ANY of what follows if you are truly following and taking consistent action on everything you've read up to this point. I truly believe that.

That's because the fundamentals of mindset, eating, and exercising that I've already taught you are really all nature needs to break through.

Consider the supplements we'll choose for you as "an added bonus". You can use them if you want, or you can skip them entirely. The only thing they might do is help you get pregnant faster. But, I believe you can get pregnant without them.

How Supplements Function As "Signal Amplifiers"

Earlier I discussed with you the concept of "Seed Intelligence".

Seed Intelligence is a term I use to describe the concept that fertility is innate, and it is constant. It is never weak or absent.

It is like a signal being broadcast from a radio tower. The signal is constantly there, always sending its information and instructions on how to create life.

How do I know it's always there? Because life will always regenerate itself, it will always seek growth and renewal.

You can't "see" Seed Intelligence, only its effects.

- A field that was brown and dried up gets a couple minutes of rain and is suddenly green and lush.
- A body tired and ravaged by cancer that recovers and is once again strong and vital.
- A single cell (egg) becoming an entire human being.

The point I'm trying to get across is this: We don't have to "put fertility inside your body", we simply must awaken and amplify the signal that's already there and give it the space to operate.

I wish I could tell you it was more complicated than that, but I can't.

I was having a conversation with my mom one day about what I do. She - like all moms - was beaming with pride. "I don't know how you do it, Chris... There are 10,000 reasons why people don't get pregnant. Yet, you make it sound so easy."

Then I said something for the first time. You know how sometimes you say stuff that even you didn't know you knew?

I said, "Yes, there may be 10,000 reasons people don't get pregnant. But there's only ONE reason they do. And that reason is that nature was able to complete the process inside their bodies."

And, it's true. That's all I've been focused on since I discovered and formulated the concepts and methods in this book which are all about ONE thing...

Helping nature do what it already knows how to do.

Instead of trying to "fix" a "condition" (aka "PCOS", "DOR", "Endometriosis", etc.), we're strengthening nature and clearing the path for it to operate. Then the body fixes itself.

Simple as that.

And as you've heard in the stories I've shared - which are just 21 of over 2000 stories I've personally witnessed at this point - it has worked very, very well.

The Problem Of Over-Complicating It

I see people all the time who come to me for help and bring with them these incredibly complicated lists of supplements. Sometimes they're literally taking 15 different supplements – that's not pills, that's 15 individual supplements.

So, if they're taking 15 individual supplements, they might be taking one, two, or three pills from each bottle and that can start to add up fast.

In fact, one of my patients was taking 48 pills every day when we first met.

Here's the good news – taking supplements that aren't really giving you benefit isn't going to kill you. It's not like pharmaceutical drugs where if you take an extra blood pressure pill or too much aspirin you can seriously hurt yourself.

The not-so-good news is that if you're taking a bunch of supplements you don't need, you might be negating the effects of the supplements you do need.

Let's take a common example I see all the time.

A lot of women will take supplements like Milk Thistle or Alpha Lipoic Acid because they were told it would help with liver function.

These two supplements, along with others out there, are very effective for activating detoxification pathways in the liver. They help speed up liver clearance of toxins.

But, people forget that the liver doesn't only clear toxins. Another important job the liver does is to help the body maintain proper hormone and neurotransmitter levels.

So, let's say you're taking a supplement like Vitex to boost your estrogen and help your body with ovulation – and you're also taking Milk Thistle or some other liver-focused supplement. These two might cancel each other out or, at the very least, the estrogen-boosting supplement may not be working nearly as well as it would on its own.

That's because all that extra estrogen is being metabolized in the liver at a much faster rate than it would be normally. So, you end up with zero net increase in estrogen or, worse, a *decrease*.

There are literally hundreds of other examples of this, but I don't want to get into it here. One thing I've learned is that this whole thing works a lot better when we just stay focused on keeping it simple, helping nature do what it wants to do, and that's it.

The Power Of Simplicity

I can't tell you how many patients of mine finally get pregnant after I help them simplify their supplement regimen down to a core group that is focused on their needs.

As I stated above, I truly believe that's because a good number of the supplements they're taking are getting in the way so that the ones they need can't work.

There are also the cases where the patients come in and they're just taking the wrong supplements.

They read online that a study says supplement X helps, and so they take that supplement. Then they read a blog that says Y and Z supplements are good for fertility, so they add those two.

Then, a friend gives them a tip on A, B, and C supplements and before they know it they're ordering them online.

And soon enough they find themselves taking 10, 15 different supplements or 48 pills a day like the person I mentioned earlier.

What I always try to do is find the most impactful supplements and focus on those. That's because I've learned that simple is better.

The process I use to select supplements is what I call "The Perfect Supplement Blueprint". It's *not* complicated – and it's not meant to be.

That's because I've found that there are essentially 5 - that's FIVE - core functional areas that are always the root cause of their problem.

I call them *"The Five Core Factors"*.

And, what I want to emphasize here is that *we don't need to address all five*.

The Five Core Factors help you simplify so you can understand where you could benefit from some key supplements.

All you must do is find the ONE or TWO areas where your body needs the most help and focus on those.

And, once we effectively address those areas using a simple supplement regimen, the rest of the fertility-boosting process - aka "The Amplification of Seed Intelligence" - happens on its own.

The reason this simple approach works is because you aren't a machine. Your body heals. It is intelligent. So, once you give those key areas the support they need, your body does the rest on its own. It knows exactly what to do.

Janice was the mother of one of my patients. She wasn't coming to me for fertility. But, her daughter worked with me and had just become pregnant with twins after two failed IVFs.

Her daughter insisted that Janice come see me. Why? Because Janice had just checked out of the hospital after a bout of severe pneumonia and, as you'll see, she'd been in poor health for quite some time before that.

For years Janice had suffered with hypothyroidism. Despite years taking thyroid medication her hair had still thinned considerably, her energy was terrible, and she was getting sick with a cold at least once a month.

On top of this, Janice had a lot of trouble sleeping.

This latest bout of pneumonia wasn't her first - it was just her most severe. She had to be in the hospital for almost two weeks. Her daughter was very concerned at this point and, hence, the "insistence" on a visit with me.

I listened carefully to Janice's story and her constellation of symptoms. Then, using my "Perfect Supplement Blueprint" process, I was able to prescribe a basic combination of 3 supplements based on what I determined were the root causes of her problem.

Upon follow-up a couple weeks later, Janice informed me that within a few days of starting the supplements along with a simple diet routine I put her on, her energy levels were better than they had been in years.

Her sleep was also dramatically improved as she was falling asleep within 30 minutes of lying down and sleeping a solid 4 hours before waking up.

This was a HUGE improvement over before where she was taking up to 2 hours to fall asleep and waking up every 45 minutes to an hour.

Miraculous? Not really. That's simply how powerful our bodies are. That's the power of Seed Intelligence when it's given the things it needs to operate at full strength.

But, the speed at which she got better does illustrate a very important principle of how I work and why I believe what I do works so well.

See, most people - including most doctors - believe the body is dumb and can't figure out what it needs to do.

They think we've got to run a bunch of tests and micromanage every little detail of the situation to get it to heal by prescribing overly-strict diets and a ridiculously overwhelming number of supplements.

And, on top of that, they see the body as something that tends to break, to fail, to get sick.

I've found the exact opposite to be true. And, this is incredibly relevant to your fertility.

After working with thousands of people over the last decade-plus, I've found the body is extremely intelligent. It knows exactly what it needs to do to heal itself and it ALWAYS heals when we give it what it needs and get out of the way.

Micromanaging the healing process stifles it. What it needs us to do is simply facilitate the completion of the healing blueprint that's already there.

Your Body Is Always Trying To Complete The Healing Process

Your body is ALWAYS trying to heal and ALWAYS trying to help you manifest your purpose. It is ALWAYS seeking a way to gain more vitality and strength.

How do we get in the way? Well, we've already addressed the most fundamental self-limiting factors by implementing "The Three Foundations". Those would be chronic dehydration, lack of rest, and an over-excited nervous system.

Back to Janice's situation... When she first came to see me, she was already taking several supplements recommended by a wellness-oriented physician who'd run all these micronutrient assays and food allergy tests and the like.

The doctor had chosen her supplements based on these test results. And, obviously, they were way off-base.

Janice wasn't feeling better after taking them for over three months. The doctor's answer to that was something along the lines of "you have to take them for a while in order for them to work."

My experience is that when your body is getting the support it needs, it wastes no time whatsoever in healing itself - or in getting pregnant - as soon as possible.

And, when your body is functioning at a higher level, you feel that immediately.

Janice was feeling better literally DAYS after starting on the regimen I recommended based on my "Perfect Supplement Blueprint" process.

All those tests - and the thousands of dollars she spent on them - had been pointless. Why?

Because her doctor was treating a piece of paper, not her.

Everyone was so busy reading Janice's tests, they forgot to ask her how she was feeling. And, even though her thyroid tests came back "in the normal range", her vitality and quality of life were far from it.

Here's another cool thing about Janice's story. Once she started feeling better she eventually stopped coming regularly. Then, about six months later she came back because she wanted a little help with some seasonal allergy symptoms.

It was then she informed me that her hair was growing back. She walked into my office and showed me the "baby hairs", as she called them, starting to show up all over her scalp.

And, she hadn't been majorly sick during that 6-month period, either. She did have a cold at one point, but her body quickly resolved it.

Even though this is not a fertility story, it clearly illustrates just how powerful and intelligent our bodies are, and how fast they heal or, in your case, become fully fertile when we support nature's power within you.

The Five Core Factors

The Five Core Factors are the essential keys to generating perfect egg quality, a receptive and healthy uterine lining, and ultimately giving birth to your healthy baby. They are:

1. Abundant Energy Reserves
2. Clear Detoxification Pathways
3. Robust Circulation
4. Stable Metabolic Foundation
5. Calm, Resilient Boundary System

The great news is that The Three Foundations support all of these and give all of them maximum space to operate.

Yet, sometimes we need to go a little deeper, and here's why.

Everyone - you and I included - comes into this world with inherent physiological challenges. These are typically called "genetic predispositions", also called our "constitution".

You see the effects of constitution in early childhood. Some kids get asthma easily, others have a lot of tummy aches or ear aches. Some are "hyperactive", others feel tired a lot. Some are great sleepers, others wake up constantly. Some get a lot of headaches or tend to run high fevers. Others rarely get headaches or run fevers.

I could go on and on but the important thing here is that as small children and growing up into adulthood we all have these "predispositions" to have certain health challenges.

And these predispositions indicate the parts of our biology that always need extra help, regardless of what is going on.

What I've found in my practice is that for every single one of my patients there is a predisposition to have problems in one or two of the Five Core Factors.

When I help them address those areas through targeted nutrition it leads to rapid acceleration of their healing - and conceiving - process.

The reason for that is we're addressing something that has been blocked or depleted for many, many years. It's that continual "wall" that your body hits before it gets all the way to conception, pregnancy, and baby.

I think I mentioned Sarah's story before but even if I did it's worth mentioning again. Sarah couldn't stay pregnant. She'd had 5 miscarriages before she came to see me.

She was barely over 30, and the doctors were starting to recommend a surrogate. That's because they had run all the standard miscarriage panels and found nothing. Everything they tried - including baby aspirin and blood thinner injections - hadn't worked, either

After hearing Sarah's story and going through her history I saw a theme - her body's boundary system (or immune system) was not functioning well. How did I know this without running tests?

Because Sarah had always had bowel issues her whole life. Alternating diarrhea and constipation. Most of the time loose stool. She felt she was very sensitive to certain kinds of foods as well, especially spicy foods.

I explained to Sarah that all her bowel issues reflected a very distressed gut boundary and that it was likely her immune/inflammatory system was shifted just enough to where her body couldn't complete the implantation process.

A word here about implantation. It's insanely complex when we analyze it, but to the body it's very, very simple.

During embryo implantation your body simply must keep itself open to allow the embryo - which is "non-self" - to attach to you. And, it does this by "turning down" the volume on your immune system just enough to allow implantation to occur.

In every other instance, your immune system wants to attack and destroy any non-self-organism inside your body as soon as possible.

But with an embryo, it knows not to do this.

In Sarah's case, her immune system was both overstimulated and depleted from the long-term inflammation in her gut, and because of this it was not able to "turn itself down" to allow implantation to occur.

Keep in mind, this is not a "malfunction". Her body *wanted* to restrain itself from attacking the embryo (as evidenced by the outcome we ended up with), it just *couldn't*.

The solution was to support the Core Factor of a calm, resilient immune system.

We focused on strengthening her gut boundary with a couple of key supplements and, almost immediately, her bowel practically normalized. Daily bowel movements with only the *very* occasional bout of diarrhea.

Just four months later, Sarah conceived and - this time - she didn't miscarry. She delivered a healthy baby girl after a full-term, healthy pregnancy.

In the chapters that follow we'll delve a little deeper into The Five Core Factors and why each is a critical element of getting pregnant.

Setting The Foundation For Seed Intelligence – The "Core Three" Pre-Conception Supplement Blend

A lot of attention is paid to "prenatal" vitamins. But really, "prenatal" vitamins are more for once you become pregnant and may not contain what is necessary to optimize your egg quality – especially if you're having trouble conceiving in the first place.

Over a decade ago I came up with a blend of 3 supplements as a core to every fertility treatment plan at our clinic.

And, just FYI, I personally take these three supplements every single day as MY core supplementation regime because I feel awesome when I do.

Aside from how good I feel taking this combination (which I've been doing religiously for over a decade), I can report to you that I rarely suffer from the common cold or flu, despite being a clinician who is routinely exposed to various cold and flu viruses here in my clinic.

First Things First: Do We Really Need These?

I'm going to be very honest here. Most people in developed countries who eat 3 meals a day probably don't "need" to take prenatal or even pre-conception vitamins.

To me, when someone asks me "do I need this?" I'm going to think in terms of, "Is this *really* something essential to their life, that they can't live without?"

Obviously, when we're talking about the supplements I'm about to tell you about, the answer is… "Of course not."

I mean, let's be real… In the United States, anyway, most of us are overfed. At the end of the day, whether we take vitamins or not we're going to be relatively OK.

Add to this the fact that there are millions of babies born every year all over the world to women who never took or much less heard of a thing called "pre-natal vitamins", and… well… you get my point.

All that being said, if you're reading this book then I am going to assume you want to do whatever you can to optimize and maximize what nature is doing to grow and produce a healthy, beautiful egg that is full of energy and ready to carry out its mission of becoming a baby.

So, these Core Three (and all the supplements that follow) represent a little "extra effort and insurance" that all your baseline nutritional components are not just bare-minimum, but the amount needed for you (and your eggs) to *thrive*.

Why The Core Three Pre-Conception Supplement Blend Is So Awesome

One of the things I like about this blend is that everything is food-based.

Food-based vitamins don't have to be dosed as high because they are in a "native" state that your body understands and, therefore, they are much more well-absorbed than synthetics.

In fact, synthetic vitamins – much like synthetic drugs – often cause unwanted (and completely unnecessary) side-effects like stomach upset, over-stimulation or sedation, changes in bowel function, sleep disturbances, and others.

It is for this reason that sometimes, in clinic, new patients are reluctant to try our Core Three.

And I assure you that, once they do start on this simple daily regimen, they almost never go back.

The reason for this is not only that they're food-based, which amplifies their effects yet with a gentleness that is unmatched.

It's also because I specifically chose these three together because they represent a "complete spectrum" that gives every Core Factor the baseline nutrients it needs.

A Quick Note

You're going to see as we go through the next few chapters that I don't mention the specific brands of supplements we use.

Bottom line is that, yes, we have very specific brands we recommend at the clinic. However, I won't be mentioning them here in the book for a couple of reasons.

1. I recognize this book is going to be traveling around the world and a lot of things we use at The Axelrad Clinic simply aren't readily available outside the United States. So, I've put

together, as best I can, a "Worldwide Egg Quality Supplement Guide" inside Axelrad Clinic Academy (which again, you can join free here: https://axelradclinic.com/awaken).

2. From time to time companies discontinue various formulations and we have to replace them. I'd rather not have to publish a new edition of the book every time that happens.

3. Trademark and other laws are just complex and after consulting with attorneys I've determined it's better to leave out the specific products and names just to be "on the safe side", legally speaking.

All this being said, I do everything I can to give you the most specific guidance possible because, fact is, quality, dosing, and potency between different supplement brands varies widely.

If I told you and another patient of mine to get a "wide-spectrum B-Complex" on your own, more than likely you would each end up buying two totally different brands and, as you might guess…

We would see two totally different responses.

One of you might complain of headaches or jitters. And, upon examining it I would discover that, indeed, the doses in the supplement were way beyond what we need.

Upon examining the ingredients of what the other of you purchased, there's a high likelihood we'd discover all kinds of added stuff like herbs, random other vitamins, and possibly fillers that we don't really want.

So, to solve this problem at the clinic, I decided I would choose the "medicines" myself (and don't fool yourself, food is powerful medicine) so I could be 100% sure not only of the quality but what response to expect at what dose.

As history has proven based on the results we get in clinic, it was a very good decision.

I'd strongly recommend you use the exact formulations we do in our clinic. And, if you can't acquire these exact brands, I'll do my best to have a list of acceptable substitutes for you in Axelrad Clinic Academy.

"Core Three" Supplement 1 – A Food-Based Wide-Spectrum Multivitamin

This has been the foundation of our supplement protocols since 2006.

Because we use a food-based multi, I've only ever heard 2 or 3 patients say it caused any kind of side-effect whatsoever (and to be honest in those cases it's debatable if the vitamin was the issue).

Dosing varies among brands but the one we use is dosed at 1 tablet daily. I usually take mine first thing in the morning on an empty stomach.

If the one you purchase doesn't have excessive amounts of B-vitamins or "energy herbs" added to it, it shouldn't disturb your sleep so it's fine to take it in the evening if you need to.

Here are the exact nutrient levels in the multivitamin we use. Keep in mind, these are food-extracted so in some cases the dose may appear low, but the potency is very, very good.

Vitamin A (Carrots*; 100 mg) -As Alpha & Beta Carotene with Mixed Carotenoids (Cryptoxanthin, Lutein, Zeaxanthin, Lycopene) - 5000 IU
Vitamin C (Oranges*; 240 mg) - 60 mg
Vitamin D3 (S. cerevisiae*; 8 mg) - 400 IU
Vitamin E (Brown Rice*; 60 mg) - 15 IU
-Tocopherols (d-alpha, d-beta, d-gamma, d-delta)

-Tocotrienols (d-alpha, d-beta, d-gamma, d-delta)
Vitamin K (Cabbage*; 7 mg) - 65 mcg
Thiamine (B1) (S. cerevisiae*; 20 mg) - 5 mg
Riboflavin (B2) (S. cerevisiae*; 50 mg) - 5 mg
Niacinamide (S. cerevisiae*; 80 mg) - 20 mg
Vitamin B6 (S. cerevisiae*; 30 mg) - 6 mg
Folate (Broccoli*; 40 mg) - 400 mcg
Vitamin B12 (S. cerevisiae*; 3 mg) - 15 mcg
Biotin (Brown Rice*; 60 mg) - 300 mcg
Pantothenate (S. cerevisiae*; 40 mg) - 10 mg
Calcium (S. cerevisiae*; 40 mg) - 2 mg
Iron (S. cerevisiae*; 90 mg) - 4.5 mg
Iodine (S. cerevisiae*; 5 mg) ⌐ 75 mcg
Magnesium (S. cerevisiae*; 40 mg) - 2 mg
Zinc (S. cerevisiae*; 120 mg) - 6 mg
Selenium (S. cerevisiae*; 25 mg) - 25 mcg
Copper (S. cerevisiae*; 10 mg) - 100 mcg
Manganese (S. cerevisiae*; 24 mg) - 1.2 mg
GTF† Chromium (S. cerevisiae*; 23 mg) - 45 mcg
Molybdenum (S. cerevisiae*; 10 mg) - 20 mcg
Potassium (S. cerevisiae*; 708 mg) - 4 mg
Boron (S. cerevisiae*; 50 mg) - 500 mcg
Phenolics* -Orange, Wild Blueberry & Cranberry
70 mg

"Core Three" Supplement 2 – A Gentle, Food-Based *B-Complex*

In my opinion, most B-Complex supplements are WAY too aggressive in their dosing. The rationale is that the body can't store B vitamins so just throw as much in there as possible and hope something sticks.

And, with synthetics that may be true.

But, a highly-absorbable (i.e. food-based) B-complex doesn't require high doses.

Additionally, high-dose B-complexes can often be overstimulating and cause some mild jitteriness or anxiety.

The B-Complex vitamins are essential cofactors for just about every essential metabolic and energy-producing process in the body.

Additionally, they are critical for nourishing and sustaining core neuroendocrine glands deep within the brain as well as the adrenal glands – which have a huge role to play in supporting the hormonal pathways that lead to healthy eggs.

So, taking a gentle Food-Based *B-Complex* is a great way to ensure ALL our cells have all the reserve energy they need on a daily basis to do what they need to do to for optimal whole-body function AND at the same time give our neuroendocrine system the "fuel" it needs to make and secrete the hormones critical to the egg development and maturation process.

Dosing of the one we use is 1 tablet in the morning, and here are the nutrient levels:

Thiamin (B1) (thiamine HCl with Cerevisiae) - 9 mg
Riboflavin (B2) (with organic brown rice) - 9 mg
Niacin (niacinamide with S. cerevisiae) - 45 mg
Vitamin B6 (pyridoxine HCl with S. cerevisiae) - 10 mg
Folate (folic acid with broccoli) 400 mcg DFE (240 mcg folic acid)
Vitamin B12 (cyanocobalamin with S. cerevisiae) - 50 mcg
Biotin (with organic brown rice) - 30 mcg
Pantothenic Acid (d-calcium pantothenate with organic brown rice) - 30 mcg
Organic Kale- 125 mg

"Core Three" Supplement 3 – A High-Quality Fish Oil Infused with Vitamin D3

The omega fatty-acids are an important part of any base pre-conception supplementation regime, as has been demonstrated by the extensive scientific research on the matter.

These fatty acids not only support brain and central nervous system function (which, again, are the core regulating system for hormonal signals), they also help the body control excess inflammation and provide important building blocks for cell membranes and other important tissue components.

Then, there's Vitamin D, which is now considered to be a critical nutrient for egg quality – so much so that IVF clinics routinely test the levels and supplement them if they come back low.

Dosing of the exact supplement we use in clinic is 2 gel caps in the morning. It's fine to take them on an empty stomach but some people do need to eat a little food with them, as the oils can require a little more "digestive juice" so to speak.

With the supplement we use, complaints about fishy smell or aftertaste are extremely rare and patients routinely refill it without question.

Here's the nutritional info on that one:

Vitamin D3 (cholecalciferol) - 1000 IU
Total Omega-3s - 1280 mg
EPA (Eicosapentaenoic Acid) - 650 mg
DHA (Docosahexaenoic Acid) - 450 mg
Other Omega-3s - 180 mg
Oleic Acid (Omega-9) - 56 mg

The exact supplements we use are available via a link from Axelrad Clinic Academy. Visit https://axelradclinic.com/awaken to learn more.

Common Questions And Answers

My doctor gave me a prenatal and I'd rather just take that. Is that OK?

Again, there's not really a "right" or "wrong" answer here. As I said above, nobody really NEEDS these things.

At the same time, based on our experience where we've helped literally thousands conceive, many of whom were not getting pregnant before switching to our blend, I never discourage someone from switching.

You literally have nothing to lose.

Will I get the recommended amount of folic acid?

Yes. If your chosen Multi + B-Complex add up to the 800mcg of recommended folic acid, in the form of folate.

Is the extra B-Complex going to hurt me or baby?

In my experience treating thousands of cases, there is zero harm and, in fact, appears to be massive benefit, from taking the extra B-Complex.

And, again, if you choose a gentle, food-based B-Complex as suggested (not one of these "Super-B" formulations trying to get you all jacked-up to run through a brick wall or something) then all you are doing is giving your body a little extra B to help it create more energy and manage your hormones more efficiently, and create the neurotransmitters it needs, and all of that simply adds up to a higher level of function on so many levels.

I'm vegetarian and can't take fish oil. What's a good alternative?

Honestly, we don't carry a vegetarian alternative but from what I understand the Omega Fatty Acids in algae-derived supplements are great, and Flax Oil has been a fundamental plant source of essential omegas forever.

And, REMEMBER...

You don't have to memorize or become an expert in any of this stuff we're about to go over.

I've got you covered in terms of how to optimize things if you just follow the process and instructions in this book and complete your *Perfect Supplement Blueprint* which is covered later.

Also, I want you to keep in mind that all the "core factors" depend on each other. Your body needs reserve energy to detoxify itself, to circulate the blood, to keep metabolism stable, and to calm any excess inflammation.

It also needs to circulate blood so that it can maintain stable metabolism, keep itself from becoming excessively inflamed, build up energy reserves, and detoxify itself.

None of these factors exists in isolation and strengthening one strengthens them all. That's the cool thing about this.

So, let's begin.

Chapter 12 - Core Factor One: Abundant Energy Reserves

Your body continually depends on its energy reserves to maintain every single body process.

These energy reserves allow your body to do what it wants, when it wants. If it needs to produce more of a hormone, it can do it right then. If it needs to warm itself up or cool itself down, or push more blood to a certain area, it can access the energy needed to do those things, too.

When your energy reserves are compromised or under too much stress, your body has difficulty responding to the moment-to-moment demands of daily life. The result is it can't do what it wants to do when it wants to do it.

In terms of your egg quality it means that resources will be diverted away from the egg-building process in order to serve a more important survival needs like managing blood pressure, fighting off infections, maintaining mental focus during times of stress, and others.

For this first core factor, your adrenal glands are the key. They are primary glands that manage and coordinate your energy reserves.

They are the foundation of your body's circadian rhythm or 24-hour body clock, which is central to every other hormonal rhythm in your body. If your circadian rhythm is altered or shifted too far outside its natural flow, every single other hormonal system will start to shift as well, including estrogen, progesterone, and testosterone as well as Growth Hormone.

The adrenal/energy reserves also impact the immune system and - if your adrenal system is depleted - you can experience immune-related issues like chronic inflammation, delayed or insufficient tissue repair, and frequent colds.

Your adrenal system also regulates your blood sugar levels between meals, keeping them stable. If this function starts to fail, you can experience weight gain (especially around the midsection), constant or intermittent bouts of fatigue, and poor sleep.

Ironically, you need reserve energy to stay asleep. That's because while you sleep, you can't eat (obviously), so your body draws upon the energy reserve system to fuel all its growth and healing processes during your resting hours.

It is a dramatic understatement to say the first core factor of Abundant Energy Reserves is incredibly important for egg quality and overall fertility.

Why Your Energy Reserves Are Critical for Conception and Pregnancy

Here's why your Energy Reserves - and the corresponding function of your adrenal glands - are so critical to getting pregnant:

1. Growth factors released ONLY during sleep are essential for proper egg maturation and growth, as well as the repair and maintenance of the tiny capillaries that supply blood to your eggs. Without those growth factors egg quality and circulation suffer.
2. The hormonal precursors such as DHEA, pregnenolone, and cortisol secreted by the adrenals are essential for both egg maturation and function of the uterine lining. Without those

precursors it's more difficult for your body to create the hormones needed to stimulate follicle, egg, and tissue growth.

3. The cortisol-immune axis is essential to support a calm and well-regulated inflammatory response. This ensures the egg and lining aren't exposed to and damaged by excessive inflammation. Without stable, healthy cortisol levels your body more easily loses the ability to regulate inflammation and hence create a receptive environment for egg, embryo, and fetus.

4. Stable blood sugar between meals - regulated primarily by cortisol - supplies the ovaries, follicle, uterus, and egg with consistent energy without the excessive insulin levels that can lead to PCOS and other metabolic hormonal disruptions. If your blood sugar starts wavering too much, there will be gaps in the developmental process of your eggs and lining.

5. During early pregnancy your body undergoes some very dramatic shifts and these shifts require extra energy, above and beyond your normal everyday levels. If the reserve energy isn't quite there to support these processes, your body is going to have a much more difficult time building the foundation needed to support full-term pregnancy.

How To Tell If Your Reserve Energy System Is Depleted

When your energy reserves are depleted, you'll feel a continual sense of tiredness. This doesn't have to be deep, deep fatigue. It COULD be, but it's more often a subtle sense of "low energy" or "lack of motivation".

The typical symptoms of depleted energy reserves would be at least two or more of the following:

- Always or easily feeling tired
- A pronounced "dip" in energy around 3-4pm

- Waking up feeling tired and sluggish
- Frequently catching mild colds (i.e. without fever or very low-grade fever) or often feeling "flu-like" symptoms
- Waking up frequently through the night and often having difficulty falling back to sleep
- A persistent feeling of "low" or "depressed" mood

If the above sounds like you, then on some level your energy reserves need help.

The Essential Ritual For Rebuilding and Protecting Your Energy Reserves

The essential ritual for supporting and stabilizing your body's energy reserves is a consistent 8-10 hours of sleep at night.

It's interesting how many people I see in clinic who think it's normal to stay up way past 10pm every night watching TV or working on their computers, routinely getting only 6 or 7 hours of sleep a night.

The bottom line is that your biology is hard-wired to sleep at night. This is not optional. Your body will support you in staying up through the night, if that's what you want to do.

But, there is a biological switch naturally begins to flip at sundown. It's the switch of melatonin and the waning of cortisol - and the entire cascade of other changes - that slow your metabolism, cool your temperature, and prepare you for a night of restorative, healing rest.

When you support your body's natural flow into sleep around 9 or 10pm, you remove an incredible amount of biological stress on your cells, glands, and tissues. In fact, you can't even imagine how much stress that one change will eliminate.

And, by getting that extra sleep you'll feel a lot more focused and energetic during the day meaning you'll get more done and have less "need" to stay up working extra hours.

My recommendation, which I outlined in The Three Foundations Of Perfect Egg Quality, is go to bed no later than 10pm every single night, preceded by a "wind-down" period - free of TVs, computers, and other electronics - of around 15-30 minutes.

Essential Supplements For Rebuilding and Protecting Your Energy Reserves

There are THREE key supplements that I've found extremely effective for rebuilding energy reserves. You don't have to take both, but you can if you wish.

Energy Reserve Replenishing Supplement 1 – Royal Jelly

So, if energy is critical to optimal growth and function of the egg, Royal Jelly is going to be a very important supplement for us to consider.

I like to think of the foods nature makes as a "language", in a sense. Certain foods are designed by nature to elicit a specific response in the parts of nature that consume that food... Just like certain words we say can certain different responses in the people who hear them.

Take fruit, for example. I believe it was mentioned earlier in the book, but if you think about fruit it is a summer food. It grows abundantly in the summer months (whether tropical or at more temperate latitudes). It's cool and refreshing and full of water. It has key minerals to replace those lost in sweat (after all, it's hot in the summer). And, it's high in sugar which, if we're on a long walk or working outside in the hot summer sun, will keep us going through the day.

Thinking of food this way, when we look at Royal Jelly, we've got some very interesting properties that make it a great choice for egg quality.

Royal Jelly is a sticky substance made by honey bees. The interesting thing about it, though, is that it is only consumed by the queen bee – hence the name "Royal Jelly".

The worker bees – and in a big hive there are tens of thousands of them – are busy literally round the clock collecting pollen, building and maintaining the nest, protecting the queen, and making honey which is used to feed the colony EXCEPT for the queen and the baby bees.

Once a larva is selected to be queen, it is exclusively fed "Royal Jelly" from that point forward for the rest of its life. It is the only bee that can consume the Royal Jelly in this manner as an adult.

The only other bees that are fed Royal Jelly are the baby bees for the first 3 days or so of their lives. After that, they consume honey like all the other bees.

The Royal Jelly, fed to the queen, is essentially a "super-food" that triggers the changes in her body that allow her to produce literally 1500 or so eggs every single day.

Royal Jelly, then, is designed by nature to convey massive amounts of energy and life-creating power to the queen bee, as well as a powerful shot of concentrated growth to baby bees during the first few days of life.

I've used it a lot in clinic. And, it never disappoints. It's a powerful nutrient but, more than that, I believe it "speaks" to the cells of our bodies with a message of growth and regeneration.

This makes Royal Jelly a very powerful substance for tissue growth and healing which, if you've been paying attention, is exactly what we want your eggs to do… We want them to GROW and STAY HEALTHY (i.e. continually heal themselves).

Now… I'm not saying you'll produce 1500 eggs by taking Royal Jelly. But, what I AM saying is based on my own clinical experience, it's a powerful superfood for egg quality because it is such a dense, concentrated energy source and, in nature, it is used specifically for reproductive purposes.

The potency of the product we use in clinic is 1500mg per capsule and typically I'll have patients take 2 capsules every morning if we're trying to support weakened or compromised Energy Reserves.

Honestly, it's a very safe nutrient but there is one warning I must mention. **If you are allergic to bees do NOT take this supplement.** It can trigger a serious allergic reaction.

In all my time I've only seen this kind of allergic reaction occur once, so they are extremely rare. But still, I wanted to mention it.

Energy Reserve Replenishing Supplement 2 – Ashwagandha

Ashwagandha is an herb from the traditional Indian medical system of Ayurveda. And, I've found it to be one of the best adaptogens - as good as or better than Ginseng in many cases.

Adaptogens are interesting compounds. They have been demonstrated to increase function that is too low, and to decrease function that is too high. In other words, they do different things depending on what your body needs.

This is because herbal medicines literally "speak" to the body. Plant intelligence and human cellular intelligence have the same source. When you ingest a plant - in particular one of the adaptogens - a "conversation" ensues, and your body intelligently responds.

This is different than with vitamins or drugs.

Vitamins are like building blocks and your body will use them as needed and try to ignore what it doesn't need.

Drugs are like commands that your body is not allowed to ignore. They will force your body to do something even if your body is barely able to do it. Therefore, they have side-effects - they'll push your body past its own limits, and you feel that as unwanted symptoms.

If your energy reserve symptoms are relatively mild, start with the Royal Jelly and, if that doesn't do the trick, add the Ashwagandha.

The product we use at The Axelrad Clinic has the following formulation. We find it to be a very gentle, effective mixture.

Sensoril®† Ashwagandha Root & Leaf Extract (Withania somnifera) - 250 mg

Rhodiola Rosea Root Extract (Rhodiola rosea) - 200 mg

Astragalus Root (Astragalus membranaceus) - 150 mg

Holy Basil Leaf (Ocimum sanctum) - 150 mg

Schisandra Berry (Schisandra chinensis) - 100 mg

Additional Foods & Extracts (Indian Gooseberry (Amla Fruit), Seaweed (Laminaria digitata and Ascophyllum nodosum)) - 145 mg

Energy Reserve Replenishing Supplement 3 – DHEA

There's controversy with this one, and for good reason.

DHEA is a hormone and, as such, it's powerful. So, I'm going to cover it here, but I must say that I would recommend you proceed carefully with this supplement, if it's even available for purchase where you live (in the USA it is available over-the-counter but in many other countries it is not).

There are situations where DHEA can cause more harm than good in terms of egg quality. So, it's important to know what those situations are, and this book can't get into every single one of them.

The two most common situations where you should avoid self-prescribing are:

1) A past (or current) diagnosis of PCOS.
2) Any blood test result showing high testosterone levels for a female.

In either of these cases, it's probably best you avoid this supplement unless instructed to take it by a medical professional, preferably your Reproductive Endocrinologist.

If you are going to self-prescribe this supplement…

…I strongly recommend you consult a qualified healthcare professional, OR make sure you start at a low dose (no more than 25mg daily) for a little while and watch for signs of excess before adding another 25mg, gradually increasing to 75mg daily if you can. I would not recommend dosing any higher than this on your own.

Signs of DHEA overdose include such things as nausea, headache, rash, diarrhea, increased blood pressure, insomnia, and heart palpitations.

These side effects are rare. But, they must be mentioned and taken seriously. If they do occur, then stop taking DHEA immediately and consult a healthcare professional before starting again.

Where I see this supplement make the biggest impact on both egg count and quality is in cases of Diminished Ovarian Reserve or low AMH where there is no previous history of PCOS or high testosterone levels.

Typical dose in my clinic for "therapeutic" purposes is 25mg morning, afternoon, and evening for a total of 75mg daily.

How To Know Your Energy Reserves Are Recovering

This is actually very simple. You'll know your energy reserves are starting to recover when you notice one or more of the following changes:

1. Start waking up in the morning with more energy.
2. Start sleeping more soundly and waking up less often. Even when you do wake up, you're less likely to stay awake for long.
3. You feel a steady foundation of energy throughout the day (doesn't mean you never get tired, you just don't feel that continual underlying tiredness anymore).
4. Your low mood days are less frequent.
5. You're not catching those mild colds or feeling run-down nearly as often.

All of these are signs your energy reserves are coming back - and with them your egg quality, lining, and ability to stay pregnant will also increase dramatically.

Chapter 13 - Core Factor Two: Clear Detoxification Pathways

Your body needs to be able to make clear decisions on what stays and what goes. That way it continually regulates the levels of hormones and other substances in the blood so that the intricate hormonal dance of the fertility/menstrual cycle happen smoothly.

When your body can make clear decisions, your body asks for more of the things it needs when it needs them and gets rid of things it doesn't need when it no longer needs them. If it wants more estrogen, for instance, it knows this and can send the signals that stimulate estrogen production. If it wants less estrogen, it can deactivate and then remove estrogen from the bloodstream.

A key component of this decision-making system of your body is its ability to release or deactivate hormones and other substances it no longer wants or needs via natural detoxification pathways in the gut and the liver.

When these natural detoxification pathways are compromised or under too much stress, your body has difficulty knowing when it needs more of something or when it needs less of something. The result is it will tend to build up excesses of certain things and create deficiencies of other things.

In terms of your egg quality it means that estrogen levels may rise and fall erratically or stay elevated longer than necessary - meaning that follicle and egg development aren't happening as smoothly as nature intended.

Think of a plant. A plant needs only so much water. If you over water it, the plant will be just as stressed as if you don't give it enough water. And, that stress is reflected as abnormal growth - either the plant withers or the plant swells. If the situation is not corrected, the plant will go on being unhealthy and may even die.

This is what happens to your eggs and lining when the estrogen levels are not properly regulated due to your body making unclear decisions.

Your liver is the primary organ that manages and coordinates these decisions in your body.

If your liver is congested or is not getting enough blood flow, it is not able to accurately sense the hormonal environment and either holds on to too much estrogen or lets go of too much too quickly. The former is what is commonly called "estrogen dominance", where estrogen levels are continually, slightly elevated. The latter is a state called "over-methylation" where your liver is going too fast and the estrogen can't rise to a sufficient level to produce a healthy egg.

Your liver also plays a role in regulating your insulin, cholesterol, and other important substances related to metabolism and tissue growth. When the liver is not functioning well, you'll potentially experience ups and downs in energy, and maybe even develop mild insulin resistance.

It's a little-known fact outside the medical community that metformin - a widely prescribed drug for PCOS and insulin-resistance - works primarily in the liver.

In other words, it tells your liver to let go of all that insulin. And, for many PCOS patients metformin - and metformin alone - shifts the entire balance in favor of conception and pregnancy for PCOS patients.

Another primary detoxification pathway for hormones is your bowel. We'll discuss that more in a later chapter.

Why Clear Detoxification Pathways Are Critical For Conception and Pregnancy

Here's why clear detox pathways - and the corresponding function of your liver - are so critical to getting pregnant:

1. Proper levels of estrogen, testosterone, prolactin, FSH, LH, and others are essential for proper egg maturation and growth, as well as for the health of supportive tissues like your nervous system and metabolic systems.
2. All these hormones must rise and fall with a certain rhythm and intensity. If the levels aren't being regulated as nature intended, it is more difficult for your body to coordinate the subtle ebb and flow necessary to produce healthy egg and lining.
3. When your detox system is blocked, not only hormones but other substances such as sugars, harmful fats, and other toxins stay in your blood and add stress to your cells and tissues, making it harder for them to do what they want to do. In other words, follicles have more difficulty growing the egg, the lining has more difficulty growing in a way that supports implantation, your immune system has more difficulty staying calm when the embryo enters the lining.
4. Not only that but the build-up of unprocessed toxins and hormonal byproducts can leak into the follicular fluid that contains the egg. As you can imagine, that creates a not-so-ideal environment for egg maturation, especially in women experiencing age-related egg quality decline.
5. When excess estrogen builds up in your system, it can also cause your blood to thicken. A big part of this thickening of the blood is initiated by your liver being overwhelmed with

too much estrogen. When your blood is too thick it can negatively affect circulation to and within your ovaries and lining.

6. During early pregnancy your body must make a lot of estrogen until the placenta can take over. If your body's ability to detoxify and remove old estrogens is impaired, it may not be getting the signal to make new estrogens, and this could affect early pregnancy in a negative way as well.

How To Tell If Your Decision-Making / Detoxification System Is Blocked

When your detoxification system is blocked, you'll feel a sense of sluggishness in your digestion, mood, and energy. You may feel heavy and bloated or have frequent bouts of nausea and headaches. You'll also tend to feel moody, irritable, and easily angered.

In severe cases, your period might become very irregular, heavy, and/or painful.

The typical symptoms of a blocked detoxification system would be at least two or more of the following:

- Feeling sluggish and heavy
- Frequent nausea and indigestion
- Regular migraines or headaches, especially around the eyes
- Feeling moody, irritable, or easily frustrated at least three or four days out of the week.
- Restless sleep and/or frequent nightmares
- Two or more of the following with your period: Heavy flow, very irregular, big clots, severe cramps.

If the above sounds like you, then on some level your detox system needs help.

The Essential Ritual For Restoring and Protecting Your Detoxification System

The essential ritual for supporting and stabilizing your body's energy reserves is to drink a minimum of 3 liters of water every day *without exception* (which is easy to do if you follow my Perfect Hydration Plan.

It's interesting how many people I see in clinic who think it's normal to drink soft drinks, bottled teas, energy drinks, flavored waters, and other processed fluids as their main source of hydration. Even more interesting is how many people I see who are chronically dehydrated and don't even realize it.

The bottom line is that plain-old, fresh, clean water is a cleanser. It cleans everything. If you look at a river flowing across rock, you will see the rock is perfectly clean, as is the water.

If the water stops flowing then stuff builds up in the water and the rock will start to look dirty or start to have algae or other things growing on it.

When you don't drink enough water, that's what happens inside your body. The flow of fluids slows down, your cells start to accumulate toxins.

Those toxins put an ENORMOUS amount of stress on your cells, but the stress on your eggs is even more significant.

I mentioned this above but it's worth repeating: As your eggs grow and develop, they are suspended inside a precious and very special drop of water inside the follicle. This water - called "follicular fluid" -

241

is a precious essence containing not only hormones but nutrition, growth factors, and, yes, cellular wastes.

If your blood is loaded with toxins your body is unable to get rid of - along with excessive hormones - the fluid inside that follicle is going to be a lot less nurturing to the egg.

The egg is already very fragile. So, every little bit we can do to help clean that follicular fluid is going to make a huge difference on how well your egg will function as a transmitter of life.

And, essentially, that's what an egg is. Remember, when you ovulate, that egg is now separate from you. It becomes the container inside which the embryo executes its first critical stages of development, relying entirely on the energy carried forward by the egg at ovulation. And it continues being a mostly self-contained entity until the placenta is fully formed.

The environment in which that egg grows - that drop of follicular fluid - is going to be the biggest determinant of whether the egg is going to struggle or thrive once it is no longer inside your ovary.

So, follow my Perfect Hydration Plan to the letter and you will be ensuring a solid foundation for that follicular fluid to be clean, pure, and full of life-giving substance.

The Essential Supplements For Restoring and Protecting Your Detoxification System

There are TWO key supplements that I've found extremely effective for restoring and maintaining healthy detoxification. You don't have to take both, but you can if you wish.

Detoxification System Support Supplement 1 – Food-Based B-Complex

I already outlined why I prefer food-based and low-dose B-Complex in a previous chapter.

The same low-dose and food-based preference applies here, and for the same reasons.

The reason B-Complex is my choice here is that the B-Vitamins are essential for healthy functioning of the liver's detoxification pathways, the synthesis of red blood cells, the maintenance of healthy cholesterol levels, and other functions in which the liver plays a key role.

Additionally, I've seen many, many cases where a little additional B Complex is enough to eliminate most if not all the symptoms of poor detoxification. Mood improves, irritability diminishes, nausea and headaches significantly reduce or are eliminated…

…just by adding a low-dose, food-sourced B-Complex.

(Yes, your body is THAT powerful when it has the right nutritional support.)

Detoxification System Support Supplement 2 – N-Acetylcysteine (NAC)

NAC is an amino acid that is a critical precursor for a very powerful organic antioxidant called glutathione (GSH).

In fact, glutathione (GSH) is, by far, the most powerful antioxidant we know of.

Your liver synthesizes glutathione, in part, from cysteine. Taking NAC helps to increase your body's bioavailable cysteine and has been shown to increase glutathione levels.

Unfortunately taking oral glutathione is a very ineffective way to raise glutathione levels because glutathione mostly degrades in the stomach and small intestine.

Why is glutathione so important? Because it - more than any other substance - helps your body to maintain healthy estrogen levels.

It is also, by the way, one of the key components in your body's natural anti-inflammatory system and is a powerful ally in your body's capacity to heal and regenerate damaged tissue.

I recommend you purchase a supplement that is pure NAC without any other ingredients. The one we use in clinic is 600mg per capsule and we generally recommend 1 capsule in the morning and 1 capsule at bedtime.

(You'll find the exact supplements we use in clinic listed in our online store, which you can access via our free portal **Axelrad Clinic Academy**. Visit https://axelradclinic.com/awaken to sign up.)

How To Know Your Detoxification Pathways Are Recovering

This is actually very simple. You'll know your detoxification pathways are starting to recover when you notice one or more of the following changes:

1. Feel that sense of sluggishness and heaviness lifting.
2. Stop having those seemingly random bouts of nausea.

244

3. Your headaches start to become much less frequent and intense (I've seen cases of chronic migraine disappear completely).
4. Excess mucus and congestion start to dissipate.
5. Your episodes of indigestion start to go away.
6. Your menstrual flow is less thick, clotty, painful and heavy.

All of these are signs your detoxification system is coming back into balance - and with it your egg quality, lining, and ability to stay pregnant will also increase dramatically.

Chapter 14 - Core Factor Three: Robust Circulatory Power

Your body needs to be able to move things towards where they need to go, and away from where they don't need to go. That way it gets the nutrients, hormones, and other vital substances to the tissues that need them and carries the natural wastes and by-products of metabolism and tissue healing away to be excreted from the body or recycled into other useful things.

When your body can maintain a constant, steady circulatory flow, tissues like your ovaries - that depend on very subtle circulatory pathways - receive the maximum amount of nutrition and hormonal stimulation possible. And, metabolic wastes (aka oxidative chemicals) are carried away efficiently.

When your body can't maintain that constant, steady circulatory flow, the hormones and nutrients simply can't get where they need to go in the quantities needed and the result is the follicles and the eggs simply won't grow as nature intended. Waste products will also build up in the local tissue in and around the ovaries as there isn't enough power to carry them away.

Even the slightest reduction of chronic inflammation or the slightest increase in tissue healing can have a dramatic positive impact on circulation, which is dependent on your most vital organ, your heart, and your most vital gland, your thyroid.

Circulation is based on momentum and space. Your heart and arteries - which really function as one organ - carry blood - a living, liquid tissue - to every single cell of your body via an intricate of tiny, tiny capillaries. Their successful, smooth movement through these capillaries depends on very subtle, but powerful variations in pulse and rhythm.

246

Your heart is continually adjusting pressure waves based on feedback from all parts of your body including brain, lungs, kidneys, and even distant tissues like the ovaries. This makes sense considering that the arteries and capillary beds are a single, connected network.

These pressure waves also react powerfully to emotional states. Background states of fear, frustration, shame, guilt, and anger lead to subtle shifts in the heart's pressure waves that make them more static and - hence - less able to respond to the needs of your body.

Imagine a symphony orchestra and a conductor. Your body is the orchestra, and your heart the conductor.

A beautiful symphonic piece is a result of a dynamic exchange between the conductor and the symphony. The conductor gives direction and pulse, and even gives cues as to the feeling and intensity with which to play certain notes. When the volume, intensity, and pulse of the music follows the subtle cues of the conductor, the result is harmonious music played as the composer intended.

But, if the conductor is not able to keep his emotional fluidity and is continually stuck on a low or high volume or a fast or slow pulse, the symphony piece starts to sound monotonous and forced.

When you're stuck on one or two subconscious emotional themes, your heart literally starts to lock into that and no longer responds to the natural ebb and flow of your cells and tissues. And, this has been shown to lead to problems like dementia, heart disease, even a higher incidence of cancer.

I guarantee that even though no research has been done to prove it, your reproductive function is dramatically affected by these same shifts in heart pulse waves.

247

Think of it this way... I'm not sure if I mentioned this earlier or not, but all your hormones are secreted in pulses. When your body wants to secrete more FSH, it makes the pulse bigger or faster. Then, it waits to see what is pulsed out by the follicle in response. Then, it adjusts the pulse based on what it thinks needs to be done.

It's a very intricate and incredibly intelligent dance of pulse and rhythm. It is, quite literally, a symphony of rhythm with thousands upon thousands of pulses overlaid upon each other.

And, the absolute core rhythm behind all of it, the first primal rhythm, is heart.

And, if heart's rhythm is not able to flow with the needs of the moment, it's absolutely going to influence the other rhythms. The timing and intensity of the pulses of FSH, LH, DHEA, Testosterone, Estrogen, and all the others will be shifted if the core pulse of the heart is shifted.

So, you're probably thinking, "OK, Chris, I get how the heart is important for circulation. But, where does the thyroid fit into all of this?"

(Before I answer that question I want to remind you that you need not be anywhere NEAR a Zen monk or enlightened being to get pregnant. So, don't worry. Just follow the simple meditations and visualizations from Part One and you'll be fine. Promise.)

Your thyroid is like the combustion chamber inside the engine of your body, and it is the most important source of energy for your heart.

Thyroid hormone is the ember that keeps your metabolic fire at an operational baseline. It's connection to the heart is unquestioned.

Your heart has been beating continuously, every single minute of every single day since you were 4 weeks gestational age. And it will continue doing so until the day you die.

It needs a lot of energy to keep that pulse going 24/7 365 - and that energy supply must be stable and consistent.

Your heart is extremely sensitive to thyroid hormone - more so than any other tissue in the body. This is why thyroid disease affects the heart so dramatically, making it beat more rapidly (excess thyroid hormone) or slowing and weakening its force (low thyroid hormone).

One more thing to note - and I find this so, so fascinating... Recently there's been a discovery that the adrenal glands secrete a hormone called "reverse T3", which effectively "turns down" the volume on the fire your thyroid stimulates.

Think of "reverse T3" as your body's way of trying to "throw a little water" on a fire that is burning a little too hot.

It's really, really interesting because I see a lot of thyroid issues in my clinic and in almost every single case I have been able to help bring about improvements by focusing NOT on the thyroid, but on the adrenal glands or, in other words, on helping my patients recover from and reduce stress.

I truly believe that "reverse T3" is a manifestation of the body knowing you need to slow down and trying to help you do just that. An overheated, overactive body can't heal and becomes chronically inflamed. That chronic inflammation starts to affect not only circulatory pathways by blocking capillaries and slowing down tissue healing, it also causes immune shifts that may lead to what we call "autoimmune thyroiditis".

In other words, if people won't slow down, the body will do what it can to make that happen - even to the point of trying to destroy parts of the thyroid, if necessary, to force us to slow down and rest.

Why Robust Circulatory Power Is Critical For Conception and Pregnancy

Here's why robust circulatory pathways - and the corresponding function of your thyroid and heart - are so critical to getting pregnant:

1. Your body won't have the energy to produce proper levels of estrogen, testosterone, prolactin, FSH, LH, and other hormones in the quantities needed if the base energy level generated by thyroid hormone isn't there.
2. The feedback mechanisms in your body that continually regulate the levels of these hormones won't get accurate information if your circulation is impaired - like a radio signal being blocked by clouds or rain.
3. When your heart is not getting enough - or is getting too much - stimulation from the thyroid, it's not able to make the subtle adjustments to pulses that are needed at various times in your fertility cycle.
4. Tissue in the uterine lining depends heavily on proper thyroid function for proper growth and function, and a natural increase in maternal thyroid hormone during pregnancy is critical for the initial development of the embryo and the ongoing growth of the fetus.
5. Circulation to the ovaries and lining is governed by a very small artery and tiny capillaries which are easily affected by subtle changes in heart pressure and rhythm.

How To Tell If Your Circulatory Power Is Diminished

The typical symptoms of shifted circulatory power would be at least two or more of the following:

- Feeling sluggish and heavy - especially in the morning.
- Swelling in the hands or feet (i.e. you wake up with swollen fingers or your fingers swell when you exercise).
- Chronically cold and/or frequently tingly hands and feet.
- Feeling significant lack of motivation or a chronic, low-grade depression.
- Mild exercise (such as walking up a flight of stairs) leading to shortness of breath with rapid heartbeat.
- Frequent heart palpitations that aren't caused by a known heart-valve problem (such as a "heart murmur").
- Two or more of the following with your period: Very light, scanty flow (i.e. only one or two days) or very heavy, prolonged flow (flow that lasts 7 days or more).

If the above sounds like you, then on some level your circulatory and thyroid systems probably need help.

The Essential Ritual For Restoring and Protecting Circulatory Power

The essential ritual for supporting and stabilizing your heart and thyroid systems is The Embryonic Breath.

As I stated earlier, your heart is your primal rhythm, and your breath is the most direct doorway to influence that rhythm.

In addition, slow, deep, rhythmic belly breathing is a literal biological switch that shifts your body out of the "stress circuit" (aka "sympathetic nervous system") and into the "relaxation circuit" (aka "parasympathetic nervous system").

251

Notice how I said "biological switch". Yes, it is that powerful and, yes, just like a light is controlled by a light switch, your body MUST go along when you practice sustained, relaxed, deep belly breathing.

When your breathing is chronically shallow your body simply cannot fully rest. When your body cannot fully rest, it can't heal. And, when your body can't heal it gets stuck in a chronic state of inflammation (which happens to be the first stage in the healing process).

That chronic state of inflammation damages the ability of your arteries and capillaries and - yes - your heart to do their job of carrying the liquid information stored in the blood to the places where it is needed.

That inflammation also has unwanted effects on your thyroid.

The good news is that your body never forgets how to heal these things and if you start now practicing your Embryonic Breath with regularity, you will guarantee yourself the best possible chance of reversing any damage, opening those circulatory pathways, and restoring smooth and stable thyroid function.

The Essential Supplements For Restoring and Protecting Your Circulatory Power

There are TWO key supplements that I've found extremely effective for restoring and maintaining healthy circulation and thyroid function. You don't have to take both, but you can if you wish.

Circulatory Power Support Supplement 1 – CoQ10

CoQ10 is an incredibly important enzyme in the process of metabolism and energy production. It is so important, in fact, that the highest concentration of CoQ10 can be found in - you guessed it - cardiac muscle tissue.

It just so happens (again demonstrating our heart - reproductive link) that CoQ10 is ALSO incredibly important for the health of arteries and microcapillaries AND is a critical nutrient in the formation and function of mitochondria.

In fact, recent studies have confirmed CoQ10 to be a powerful tool to help with improving egg quality. And, it's no wonder.

Think about this. After you ovulate, your egg essentially becomes a space capsule. It disconnects from your body and must supply all the energy needed for the ongoing growth of the embryo, then early fetus, until the placenta is fully functional and nutrient flow is fully established between you and baby.

There is a critical stage just before ovulation where mitochondria migrate from your body into the egg. They are like the little batteries that will supply energy to the space capsule until it lands on its little planet (your uterine lining) and can set up its base camp and get its food supply stabilized (the placenta).

I give CoQ10 to pretty much ALL my fertility patients. That's because most - if not all - of the people I see are, I believe, in some state of metabolic deficiency. That's either due to age or due to long-term chronic stress and less-than-ideal diet.

I also believe from my clinical experience that CoQ10 is very, very helpful for the formation of uterine lining (which is a blood vessel-rich tissue) and even helps the baby's heartbeat both directly (as a result of its presence in the yolk sac of the embryo) and later as it flows into the baby's bloodstream through the placenta.

253

I recommend Ubiquinol (which is a "micronized" and more easily absorbed form of CoQ10) at a dose of 100 - 200mg twice daily.

The Ubiquinol we use in clinic is 100mg per gel cap and for most patients 1 gel cap in the morning and 1 at bedtime is enough.

Circulatory Power Support Supplement 2 – Vitamin E + Zinc + Selenium

Vitamin E, Zinc, and Selenium are essential for healthy functioning of both thyroid and heart, and are critical supportive nutrients for arteries, veins, and capillaries.

As a bonus, all three of these nutrients also play critical roles in both ovarian and uterine function. Think that's a coincidence? I think not.

I won't go off on a major tangent here but it's important to point out that in the physiology of Chinese Medicine there is a direct, indisputable link between heart and reproductive function. This link has been stated as fact in Chinese Medicine for many, many centuries.

I find it no coincidence then, that the nutrients I mention in this chapter are key in the functioning of the heart AND the ovaries, uterus, and egg.

The formulation we use at The Axelrad Clinic has the following nutrient combination and dosage:

Vitamin A (as beta carotene) - 10000 IU
Vitamin E (as d-alpha tocopherol succinate) - 100 IU
Riboflavin (vitamin B2) - 25 mg
Zinc (as zinc picolinate) - 5 mg
Selenium (as selenomethionine) - 100 mcg
N-acetyl-l-cysteine (NAC) (free-form) - 100 mg
Milk thistle (silybum marianum) extract (seed) (standardized to contain 80% silymarin) - 100 mg

Mixed carotenoids (from lutein, lycopene and zeaxanthin) - 500 mcg

The above is the nutrient content of a single capsule. We have patients take 1 capsule in the morning and 1 (sometimes 2, depending on the situation) at bedtime.

One thing you may have noticed is the high dose of Vitamin A in the above supplement.

It's important to keep in mind that in this case (as in ALL our supplements we use at the clinic) the Vitamin A is in the form of beta carotene and as such there is no concern about toxicity.

How To Know Your Circulatory Power Is Recovering

You'll know your circulatory power is starting to recover when you notice one or more of the following changes:

1. Less or no swelling in your fingers, hands, and feet.
2. Waking up in the morning more easily.
3. Feeling cold less easily - especially in your hands and feet.
4. A general lift in your mood - not feeling "down" as often.
5. Sharper mental focus.

All of these are signs your circulatory power is coming back into balance - and with it your egg quality, lining, and ability to stay pregnant will also increase dramatically.

Chapter 15 - Core Factor Four: Stable Metabolic Foundation

Your body needs to have a stable environment in which to operate, where there aren't large fluctuations in the amount of glucose (which is essentially gasoline to the cells). That way the billions of processes happening inside the cell can continue at a steady, smooth pace, and there are minimal interruptions to the work that needs to be done at any given moment.

A stable metabolic foundation is critical to the function of your ovaries and the growth of the eggs inside the follicles. When there is stability, growth processes are smooth, consistent, and much, much more likely to produce healthy eggs.

When that stable metabolism is lacking, there are continual interruptions in the growth process of the eggs. Your body literally must "pause" the process while it deals with swings in glucose. Then, later, when it tries to pick back up on the growth process, the egg has potentially undergone damage either from the excessive glucose load or the lack of available glucose.

Even the slightest shift towards stability can have a dramatic positive impact on your egg quality and ability to conceive. While many would say this stability is tied to your pancreas and insulin, it really isn't. True, your pancreas secretes insulin, but it is only reacting to the sugar you are consuming.

So, at least in my view and experience, the balance of this core factor depends almost entirely on the amount of sugar you are eating.

And, I'm not just talking about refined/white sugar.

One of the things I love about Chinese Medicine is how they classify foods by taste. The five tastes are sweet, sour, salty, spicy, and bland.

It would be funny if it weren't so tragic... Over 1,000 years ago, in the texts of Chinese Medicine, the following principle was clearly stated: "Too much sweet food damages the body and causes the body to store fat. When the body stores too much fat, its energy is depleted and circulation is blocked, and this causes disease to take root."

OK, they didn't say it EXACTLY like that. Instead of "fat" they said "dampness", instead of "depleted energy" they said "damaged Qi", instead of "blocked circulation" they said "blocked Qi".

But, what I said first is exactly what they meant. Too much sweet food leads to obesity which leads to every kind of disease you can think of.

Why? Because sweet foods trigger a certain biological response in the body that tells it to start creating fat. Even if the "sweet" is "artificial", the body still reacts to "sweet" with this same biological patterning.

It's why they've proven that people who drink diet sodas don't get any benefit in terms of weight reduction or obesity prevention.

Another important thing -- many foods may not taste sweet to your palate, but they quickly become sweet once they enter your system.

I talked about this as part of the Sun Cycle Diet, but it's worth noting here, too. Milk is loaded with sugar - in particular lactose - that is broken down into glucose very, very rapidly. Wheat flour is extremely high in simple sugars that rapidly spike your glucose levels as well (yes, even the brown, so-called "whole-wheat" flour).

So, it's VERY IMPORTANT to know that ANYTHING that rapidly transforms to glucose inside your body is going to cause a lot of damage - to everything, and especially your eggs and uterine lining.

Why? Well, the interesting thing here is it's not the sugar itself. The sugar is simply a "tool" for your body to use. If sugar was toxic, you'd die as soon as you ate it.

What's toxic to your body - over time - is the excessive insulin it secretes as it tries to handle all the sugar.

Insulin is the single most important hormone your body makes, bar none. It is the facilitator for cells digesting glucose that is in the bloodstream.

Because of its importance, when large amounts of insulin are secreted, EVERYTHING else pretty much stops. Think of insulin like a big fat pause button for the hormonal system.

Your eggs and follicles are cruising along, listening to the signal of how to grow a healthy egg, when suddenly the signal is completely interrupted by the insulin "emergency alert system". Everything is interrupted for a second, and healthy growth cannot continue until the alert system calms down and the healthy egg signal is once again audible.

Now, your body can easily handle small fluctuations in sugar and insulin levels, and still produce healthy eggs. It's not made of paper and it's not so fragile that the we need to become obsessive-compulsive about ridding every drop of sugar and carbohydrate from the diet.

But, the extreme levels of sugar in the modern diet - which is comprised of large amounts of processed grains, dairy, and other hidden sugars - triggers an insulin wave that is more like a tsunami. It's damaging everything in its path.

So, the key is to remove the trigger by reducing the amount of sugar consumed. Not just candy and cookies, but the hidden sugars in dairy, wheat flour, and other highly processed foods.

Why A Stable Metabolic Foundation Is Critical For Conception and Pregnancy

Here's why stable metabolism and the corresponding stabilization of insulin levels are so critical to getting pregnant:

1. Insulin makes fat cells grow. Excessive fat levels shift your body's estrogen cycle.
2. Dramatic swings in your blood sugar make it very difficult for your body's hormonal system to self-regulate because of how stressful they are for your adrenal glands and liver.
3. If high levels of sugar stay in the blood too long, it causes a tremendous amount of stress on nerves, blood vessels, and other vital tissues. Therefore, diabetics have circulatory problems, reduced immunity, swelling, and neuropathy.
4. Insulin is very similar to a very important hormone for egg maturation called Insulin-Like Growth Factor (IGF). High levels of insulin disrupt the normal function of this growth factor, hence disrupting the normal growth of eggs
5. The inflammatory state that ensues from metabolic instability shifts immune function as well, and the inflammatory chemicals can damage eggs and lining.

How To Tell If Your Metabolic System Is Unstable

The typical symptoms of unstable metabolism would be at least two or more of the following:

- Sudden heaviness or sleepiness during the day - especially within an hour of a meal OR if you haven't eaten for over 3 hours.
- Frequent episodes of dizziness, shakiness, weakness, and/or sweating accompanied by hunger.
- Frequent, sudden cravings for starchy, bready, or sweet foods.
- Bouts of nausea and/or headaches that are relieved by food.
- Waking up in the middle of the night with the urge to eat.
- Mid-section or belly fat that just won't go away.

If the above sounds like you, then on some level your metabolic system probably needs help.

The Essential Ritual For Restoring and Protecting Your Metabolic Stability

The essential ritual for stabilizing your metabolism is The Sun Cycle Diet.

As you've probably figured out, I'm big on rhythm (and it's probably no coincidence that I'm a drummer and even studied percussion in college). And, with metabolism, rhythm is as important as can be.

By eating in rhythm, you take a tremendous amount of stress off your metabolic system. And, by eating in sync with the sun cycle, you virtually ELIMINATE the stress.

That's because your body's core metabolic rhythm - the cortisol circadian rhythm - naturally aligns itself with the sun. So, when you eat in rhythm with the sun you are also aligning your nourishment with your body's core metabolic state.

Doing the Sun Cycle Diet is like pushing the "Easy Button" for your metabolism. It removes massive amounts of biological stress that do nothing but interfere with the subtle endocrine states that produce a healthy egg and baby.

The Essential Supplements For Restoring and Protecting Your Metabolic Stability

There are TWO key supplements that I've found extremely effective for restoring and maintaining metabolic stability. You don't have to take both, but you can if you wish.

Metabolic Stability Support Supplement 1 – Myoinositol

Myoinositol is commonly referred to as simply "Inositol". It is a B-vitamin-like compound that is not part of the traditional "B-complex" - that has powerful stabilizing properties for metabolism.

Inositol assists the body with the signals that control how insulin works and has a stabilizing effect on cell membranes. It is a powerful tool for helping stabilize the insulin-glucose system.

It has also been studied in the treatment of depression and other mood disorders, with favorable results even at very, very high doses. And, the higher doses did not cause any reported toxicities (don't take this as an endorsement of you gobbling large doses of inositol - I'm just pointing out it's been deemed a very safe compound).

I've seen inositol have a dramatic impact on egg quality during IVF cycles of my patients, especially those who have issues with this core factor or who are overweight. Many of them had failed one or more times and then had success as soon as they added inositol.

In the clinic, we use a pure inositol supplement that contains 900mg per capsule and we typically have patients take 2 capsules twice daily – once in the morning and once in the evening.

Quick note: Inositol should NEVER be expensive. If you're paying a lot of money for inositol, you're being ripped off.

Also, I have seen zero difference in terms of results between Myoinositol and D-Chiro Inositol at the recommended doses.

Metabolic Stability Support Supplement 2 – Chromium Picolinate

Chromium picolinate is a trace mineral, meaning your body requires very, very little of it - so be careful with this one as it is easy to overdose. It is an essential component in the transport of glucose into cells, and it is easily depleted in people who have insulin resistance.

PCOS is often associated with insulin resistance, so adding chromium picolinate just before large meals can be helpful.

Our chromium picolinate is 200mcg per capsule, and when we prescribe it, we have patients take one before each meal.

Something Important

I want to point something out: ***NOTHING SUBSTITUTES FOR HEALTHY EATING. PERIOD.***

Sure, it is possible to take these supplements - or to take a pharmaceutical drug - to override a crappy diet that is out of sync with the sun and/or full of sugar whether from candy, sweets, and cookies or an excess of dairy, fruit, and wheat flour.

However, I never recommend using inositol or chromium-picolinate to attempt to offset bad eating habits.

Use them in *combination* with *The Sun Cycle Diet* to help your body shift back to balance more quickly, then you can stop when you don't need them anymore.

How do you know you don't need them anymore? Your diet is on track and you're no longer having any of the symptoms of metabolic instability mentioned above.

How To Know Your Metabolic Stability Is Recovering

You'll know your metabolic stability is starting to recover when you notice one or more of the following changes:

1. Strong energy dips are rare or completely absent.
2. Craving for carb-dense foods is no longer an issue.
3. You no longer feel well (i.e. you'll feel significant fatigue and brain fog) after eating bread, dairy, or other high-carb low-fiber foods.
4. Any frequent, sudden episodes of shakiness or dizziness become rare or go away completely.
5. That nagging mid-section or belly fat starts to dissipate.

All of these are signs your metabolism is stabilizing - and with it your egg quality, lining, and ability to stay pregnant will also increase dramatically.

Chapter 16 - Core Factor Five: A Calm, Resilient Boundary System

Your body has a built-in protection system to keep harmful things out and let helpful things in. I call this the "boundary" and it encompasses not only your immune system but your digestive lining, your skin, your lungs, and all the internal barriers that protect precious tissues like brain, lung, retina, testis, and ovaries from the general blood circulation.

Clear, calm boundaries are critical to the health of your eggs and the function of your lining.

The follicle itself is like a boundary, keeping the highly refined essence of follicular fluid inside and separate from the general blood circulation outside.

Your lining is, itself a boundary between "self" and "not-self" - it literally contacts the "outside world", part of which is this new being called an embryo that wants to attach to you and take blood and nutrients from you.

If your body's boundary system is in some way weakened or overly stimulated, there will be excessive inflammation in your body.

Now, this is important, so I want you to remember it: Inflammation is not bad.

That's right, *I said inflammation is NOT bad.*

Inflammation is a stage in the healing process. So, when your body is injured you want it to get inflamed so it can heal.

Problems arise when your body stays inflamed for long periods of time. This results in a delayed healing process and widespread tissue damage, among other things.

So, our goal should NEVER be to suppress or eliminate inflammation, for that is suppressing the healing process (of course, there are exceptions as in severe autoimmune disease where, without suppression, organs may be destroyed causing severe pain and possibly death).

Our goal is to shore up the boundaries so they can calm down and very naturally return to baseline after the healing process is complete.

When your boundary system is overactive or depleted, your body cannot exit the inflammatory stage, and this changes the follicular and uterine environment so that it is more difficult to keep follicular fluid pure and stay receptive during implantation.

It's always worth mentioning this: Your eggs, and any embryo resulting from them (or those of an egg donor), is NOT you. Its DNA is not identical to yours.

In every other situation where an organism that doesn't match your DNA tries to enter your body, the boundary system will try to block it and kill it. Simple as that.

For instance, we know there are friendly bacteria and many other organisms living inside your gut and on your skin. But, those organisms are NEVER intentionally allowed to enter your bloodstream or exchange fluids with you in any way, shape or form. That is how the boundary is set up. Live and let live.

If any of those "friendly" organisms try to enter or attach to your blood system your body is supposed to react fiercely and ruthlessly to block and/or kill the invader immediately.

But, in the case of the embryo, your body "knows" this is your child. And, it makes an extraordinary exception.

It allows your child to attach to you, to form blood vessels that link to yours, and to be nourished by you. It even allows cells from your child to enter your bloodstream and live inside you.

It's a beautiful bonding process that only nature could orchestrate. And, science is still trying to understand the exact mechanisms of how it works.

My opinion, they'll never fully understand it because it's more than just a chemical process. There is a fundamental spiritual process at work that guides the chemicals to do what they do, and spirit is something we can't - and never will be able to - measure with scientific instruments.

So, why do drug addicts get pregnant if it's a spiritual process? Because even a drug addict has spirit. She may be in pain, suffering, and living a misguided life, but she is still spirit and if there is spirit and life and the body is producing eggs and has a uterus, it is possible for that spirit to complete its life-creation blueprint.

So, the boundary system is incredibly important to this process of creating life because it is like the gatekeeper. When your boundary system is calm and clear, it can easily discern "friend" from "foe" and hence the implantation process goes smoothly.

Additionally, your body's ability to keep clear boundaries ensures the hormones, proteins, growth factors, wastes, and other information carried in the blood can enter the places they need to enter so your entire system gets what it needs and doesn't get extraneous stuff.

For example, your brain has a barrier, too. Certain things aren't supposed to enter your brain otherwise they'd cause damage. When the boundary system is weak, your brain barrier can't keep everything out and your brain literally starts to get inflamed. This is a recently discovered phenomenon.

If your brain is inflamed, this can affect how your nervous system is regulating all the body processes involved in egg maturation, ovulation, uterine receptivity, and other critical functions. Just like any other tissue, if it's under too much stress, it's not going to function at peak capacity.

I want to re-emphasize something here because I've just said a whole lot in the preceding paragraphs that may be a little overwhelming:

Your body knows how to fix all of this, and it doesn't have to be close to perfect for you to get pregnant. Don't overanalyze or start worrying about whether your brain is inflamed.

Just follow the guidance I have given you and your body will take care of it on its own. Your body WILL heal. Promise.

Your boundary system has three primary components, as I mentioned earlier: Your gut, your lungs, and your skin.

All these tissues in some form or another are exposed to the outside world and demarcate "outside" from "inside".

Ensuring the health of these three primary components is a HUGE key to supporting clear, calm boundaries. And, it's very easy to do.

Why Clear, Calm Boundaries Are Critical For Conception and Pregnancy

Here's why clear, calm boundaries and the corresponding reduction of excessive inflammation are so critical to getting pregnant:

1. Chronic, even low-grade inflammation can disrupt growth and damage both the egg and the uterine lining.
2. An overactive immune system can deplete your reserve energy so that the resources your body needs to make hormones and proteins is shifted away from making eggs and creating healthy lining.
3. Cervical mucus is derived from gut-mediated sources, meaning that if there is inflammation in your gut, it can affect the state of this vital secretion.
4. External boundaries that are weak will lead to a higher toxic load for your liver - which not only filters your blood but also plays a critical role in regulating estrogen and other hormone levels.
5. The more your body is stressed by ongoing inflammation, the faster it ages. That's because your body can't fully restore and heal while it is in the inflammatory stage.

How To Tell If Your Boundary System Is Weak or Inflamed

The typical symptoms of weak or inflamed boundaries would be at least two or more of the following:

- Any type of chronic bowel irregularity - diarrhea, loose, constipation… with or without pain, urgency, blood, mucus.

- Chronic unresolved allergies - even upper-respiratory - for which you must take frequent antihistamines.
- Severe bloating and fullness after meals - especially if those meals include wheat flour, dairy, or other processed foods.
- Chronic skin irritations like hives, rashes, eczema, psoriasis.
- Catching cold more than once or twice a year. Also taking a long time to recover from colds - like lingering cough and congestion.
- Very clotty &/or painful periods - as this may be a sign of inflammation in the lining.

If the above sounds like you, then on some level your boundary system needs help.

The Essential Ritual For Restoring Clear, Calm Boundaries

The essential ritual for restoring and maintaining clear, calm boundaries is The Three Foundations Of Perfect Egg Quality.

If you remember, The Three Foundations are:

1. 2-3L of water daily
2. 8-10 hours of daily sleep AT NIGHT (i.e. bedtime by 10pm).
3. The Embryonic Breath

You're thinking - what does drinking water, sleeping, and breathing have to do with my gut, skin, lungs, and immune system?

The water cleanses your system of toxins that are irritants and provoke excessive inflammation as your body must continually try to deal with them.

The sleep gives your body a chance to heal. So, boundary tissues (which depend on collagen for proper function), have a chance to regenerate and strengthen under the influence of growth hormone.

The breathing calms your nervous system to shift out of the immunosuppressive "fight or flight" mode. In other words, by relaxing you allow your immune system to finish the healing process.

Is diet important here? Absolutely. It's critical. It is ALWAYS critical and regardless of which area you are working on, you should follow The Sun Cycle Diet for your eating. It is, in my opinion, one of the easiest ways to help your body on so many levels, including eliminating chronic inflammation and completing the healing process.

The Essential Supplements For Restoring and Maintaining Calm, Clear Boundaries

There are TWO key supplements that I've found extremely effective for keeping your boundary system healthy and strong. You don't have to take both, but you can if you wish.

Clear Boundary Support Supplement 1 – N-Acetylcysteine (NAC)

N-Acetylcysteine - commonly referred to as "NAC" - an amino acid that is essential for proper function of mucus membranes including lung, intestine, and sinus.

Something to note quickly here. I want you to realize that from the opening of your mouth and nose to the opening of your anus, there is a single, unified mucus membrane.

Yes, the cellular structure differs slightly as it moves through your body, but your mouth, throat, sinuses, lungs, esophagus, stomach, small and large intestine, and rectum represent an "inner skin" that is one continuous, connected membrane.

Think about that and realize that if you have had chronic gut or lung or allergy problems, you might be getting clues about why you're not getting pregnant. It tells you your boundaries could be compromised, and this could be reflected in the function of your uterine lining and the follicular boundary.

When you take NAC, it helps heal these membranes and boosts production of glutathione, the most powerful antioxidant for protecting cells against damage from the byproducts of inflammation.

I've seen NAC have what I believe is a huge impact on patients of mine with recurrent miscarriage, PCOS, and endometriosis – all of which have been correlated with high inflammatory load.

Use NAC for more general issues that are affecting both upper and lower - like upper respiratory allergies and chronic mucus and/or gut symptoms.

We use pure NAC, 600mg per capsule. I typically recommend 1 capsule in the morning and 1 at bedtime.

The reason for the dose at bedtime? Because when you sleep your liver fills with blood - so this is a great time to take this precious liver-supporting nutrient.

Clear Boundary Support Supplement 2 – Systemic Proteolytic Enzymes

Systemic enzymes are enzymes that the body uses internally to break down proteins in the blood. They're a very powerful (and essential) component of ensuring that inflammation and clotting are well-managed during the tissue healing process.

271

Ongoing excessive inflammation, especially in the gut tissue, can lead to a depletion of systemic proteolytic enzymes, making it more difficult for the body keep the boundary areas clear and calm.

I've used these compounds – and Natto-Kinase in particular – for many years in cases of recurrent miscarriage and endometriosis associated with boundary weakness. And, they never disappoint.

The one we use has the following composition per capsule, and we usually recommend patients take 1 capsule in the morning and one at bedtime:

Nattozimes (2000) FU) exo/endo proteases - 129 mg
Serrazimes (20,000 U) exo/endo proteases - 33 mg

Clear Boundary Support Supplement 3 – L-Glutamine

L-Glutamine is an amino-acid as well, and it is found in high concentrations in the intestinal membranes as well as the all-important lymph tissue which functions as a critical barrier surrounding the small and large intestine.

Use L-Glutamine ESPECIALLY if your symptoms are more lower-intestinal, such as constipation, IBS, cramping, urgency, etc. It is amazing for this.

We use a pure L-Glutamine delivered as 1000mg capsules. Our generally recommended dose is 2 capsules in the morning.

L-Glutamine is also a precursor to Glutamate which is great for energy and focus. It is for this reason I don't recommend you take it at night.

How To Know Your Boundary System Is Recovering

You'll know your boundaries are starting to recover when you notice one or more of the following changes:

More consistent well-formed stool - and daily bowel movements.
Less allergic reactivity to your environment and less need for antihistamines.
No massive abdominal bloating after meals.

- Hives, rashes, or outbreaks of eczema/psoriasis become rare or may go away completely.
- You catch cold rarely and when you do recovery is quick.
- Less clots in the period flow.

All of these are signs your boundary system is calming down - and with it your egg quality, lining, and ability to stay pregnant will also increase dramatically.

See the exact brands of supplements we use at The Axelrad Clinic in our always free Axelrad Clinic Academy.

Visit https://axelradclinic.com/awaken to sign up.

Chapter 17 - Your Perfect Supplement Blueprint

The temptation here is to just take ALL the supplements I just mentioned and "cover all the bases". That's what most people tend to do when they read stuff like this.

But, that's the worst thing you can do, in my opinion.

Again, you want to focus on the areas that need help because once those areas are strong, everything else will usually fix itself.

And, if you over-supplement you could be canceling out the effects of your most helpful supplements or, worse, causing new problems you didn't have before.

So, here's what you do:

1) Go back through the symptom lists in the previous chapters.
2) Next to each symptom, write a "0" if you pretty much never have it, a "1" if you sometimes have it, and a "2" if you have it very often or all the time.
3) After you finish this, go back and for each of the five sections, add up the total.
4) You should now have at least one, maybe two sections with the highest total score.
5) For the area with the highest score, take BOTH supplements I mentioned - this is the area that needs the most help.
6) For the area with the second highest score, take the FIRST supplement only. The first supplement is the more gentle, general option.

This will reduce the general supplement load dramatically for most people. And, in my experience, when people are putting together their own supplement regimes (even healthcare practitioners), it's best to simplify and, if you want to get more detailed, go seek the guidance of a qualified practitioner.

What to do if there is no clear "winner" on the symptom scores

Sometimes you might have three areas tied for the lead or tied for second.

In this case, I want you to trust your own judgment and pick the ONE area that has been bothering you the LONGEST.

For instance, if boundaries, reserve energy, and metabolism all score a 7, you need to think back...

Which are started showing symptoms first?

You will realize that one of them started before all the others, and *that's* the one you choose to supplement as the "highest score" area.

In this case, you would then take the other two that got a 7, and you would do the same thing. Which one of those two came first? Then supplement that one with ONLY the first supplement.

I want you to start this way, so you're not taking more than our Core Three plus three additional supplements.

The very focused supplement choices along with The Three Foundations and The Sun Cycle Diet will give you a very, very, very powerful shift towards incredibly healthy eggs and receptive lining.

Oh, and you will probably feel better than you've felt in a long, long time... Maybe even your entire life.

My patients often tell me they feel amazing as ever, and I'm not surprised because unfortunately many of us were overloaded on sugar and processed foods since we were infants and toddlers.

On top of this, many of us have had poor sleep and hydration habits for decades which is never helpful over the long-term.

Don't let this discourage you.

REMEMBER...

Your body is incredibly powerful and is the embodiment of the very creative power of nature. Given the support it needs and the opportunity to do so, it will INSTANTLY begin the process of self-restoration and regeneration.

Chapter 18 - For The Guys

There are key things we can do to ensure the male side of the equation is as healthy as possible, as well... Which is obviously important if you have a male partner.

First thing to do, if you haven't already, is to have your partner do a semen analysis and medical exam (by a urologist or qualified specialist). I'm never surprised anymore to hear a couple tell me they've been trying for over a year without any testing on either the male or female side.

The reason I recommend an exam by a urologist or specialist is just to rule out things ahead of time. Just like on the female side, there are a lot of conditions that have no symptoms yet may have a significant impact on fertility.

A qualified specialist will be able to rule those out easily upon physical examination.

Also, I strongly recommend you do semen analysis at a fertility clinic or, at the very least, make sure you ask the physician offering to perform the test if they use a certified andrology lab.

Believe it or not, semen analysis is still a manual endeavor. In other words, it consists of a human simply looking through a microscope, counting stuff, and visually inspecting the shape and movement of the sperm.

In other words, you want someone with experience doing that, to make sure you get the most accurate result possible.

And, this brings me to another point that's important to point out.

277

A semen analysis is not a fertility test.

True, by looking at sperm under a microscope we can see whether they look reasonably healthy, if they have enough numbers, and are capable of swimming straight (or at all).

But, none of these parameters tell you for sure if the sperm cells themselves are going to be able to successfully fertilize an egg.

So, just because your partner is told they have "Superman" sperm because of high concentration, good motility, and what appears to be normal shape...

...if your partner has never had children prior to this, a high-grade on a semen analysis is pretty much meaningless for the purposes of determining outcome.

Just FYI.

It's better than finding out your partner has little to no sperm in the semen, which *does* indicate very low to zero likelihood of pregnancy without In-Vitro Fertilization (IVF).

Obviously the arena of male fertility is complex, and we could start a whole new book on it right here. But, it's not my intention to do that.

In Axelrad Clinic Academy I've got links to articles and other resources for you to go into more detail, should you desire to do so.

For now, what I'm going to focus on is making sure we've got all the basic things covered to ensure the best possible outcome for you.

First Things First...

Everything I've already covered in this book applies just as much to the male side as the female side. So, anything your partner is willing to do in the realms of sleep, hydration, diet, mindset, and supplementation that is outlined here is great.

Secondly, when it comes to the male side of the equation things are just a lot simpler.

As we all know, the female fertility cycle – the beginning (or end, depending on your perspective) of which is marked by menstruation - takes place over a period of around 3-6 weeks.

Incidentally, this means that, for the most part, a woman's hormones are different every single day of her life starting with puberty all the way until menopause.

The male fertility cycle, on the other hand, is 24 hours.

Yep, that's right. A man's hormonal pulses are pretty much the same every single day. And, a healthy male will make literally millions of sperm (sometimes upwards of 100 million) during that 24-hour period.

This is a good thing when it comes to helping the male side because, again, it simplifies things quite a bit.

Still, there are things we want to pay attention to in order to ensure things are as optimal as possible with the sperm.

Temperature

The testes are located outside the body cavity because sperm must grow in an environment that is below normal body temperature.

Therefore, anything that may heat up the testes on a continual or even periodic (but regular) basis need to be examined and, if necessary, changed.

These things would include:

1) Wearing tight underwear that presses the testicles up against the body.
2) Any type of compression of the testicles such as when riding a bicycle for long distances.
3) Frequent use of hot tubs, saunas, steam rooms.
4) Frequent taking of hot baths.
5) Working even for just a few hours a day with a laptop computer sitting directly on the lap.

So… if any of the above situations are in play, feel free to address them. Wearing loose underwear such as boxer shorts, ceasing long-distance cycling, minimizing saunas, hot tubs, and hot baths, and keeping that laptop on a table or desk are all good basic practice.

Testosterone

In terms of male fertility, testosterone functions much like estrogen, guiding the maturation and growth of the sperm to ensure they are ready to do their job.

Therefore, it's important to make sure testosterone levels are at least decent to ensure good sperm function.

Things that can hinder ample testosterone levels include:

1) All the stuff under temperature (because those high temperatures hinder the cells that produce testosterone).

2) Being overweight or obese – especially with high amounts of belly fat – can suppress testosterone levels because fat cells convert testosterone into estrogen.

3) Lack of quality sleep can cause problems with testosterone because, just like with females, hormones critical to the male fertility cycle are only secreted at night during sleep.

4) Poor stress management can be an issue because, as with the female cycle, excessive cortisol can have a detrimental impact on testosterone production.

And, finally, I want to make special mention of this:

A male who wants to conceive a child must never take testosterone supplementation. Ever.

It's basically male birth control, as when a man supplements testosterone his body slows or stops its production and – with that – the sperm-making process also slows or stops.

I've seen cases where the male partner is given testosterone as a treatment for low energy or low libido or simply because he tested with low levels, and the couple tries to conceive for months without realizing he is pretty much infertile the entire time.

If your partner is currently supplementing testosterone make sure you consult with a physician about the safest way to stop. Depending on the dose there can be some issues coming off.

Stress

Again, here we're talking not just about "life stress" but biological stress that impacts sperm health.

The dietary and lifestyle principles in this book go a long way to helping anyone minimize both emotional and biological stress, so as stated earlier if your partner is willing to implement these things that's always a good idea.

Other things to watch out for in terms of biological stress on sperm include:

1) High caffeine consumption (more than 1 serving per day)
2) High alcohol consumption (more than 1-2 servings per week).
3) Excessive marijuana use (again, more than 1-2 times per week).
4) Low protein, low-fat, high-carb diets.
5) High chemical exposures without proper protective measures (i.e. regularly working with volatile chemicals, pesticides, etc.).

Key Supplements For Sperm Health

The Five Core Factors as outlined before are a great starting point for choosing specific supplements for the male side of things. So, if you want to go that route and have your partner complete the process of determining his two most dominant factors that need help, go for it.

However, there are some general supplements that help with the male side of things regardless of the situation so if you want the "easy button" we can go that route, too. Up to you.

Sperm Support Supplement 1 - High-quality Food-based Multivitamin

This is always the foundation. So, don't overlook it.

I go over the exact formulation we use at The Axelrad Clinic in Chapter 11 in the section about our Core Three Pre-Conception Supplements.

Sperm Support Supplement 2 - A Wide-Spectrum Antioxidant containing Vitamin E + Zinc + Selenium

Number two on our "general sperm health" supplement list is a wide-spectrum antioxidant.

Again, the one we use, which is detailed It's a very nice mix of Vitamins A (beta-carotene) & E, Zinc, and Selenium – all of which are good for sperm and help protect the sperm from excessive oxidative chemicals.

The formulation we use at The Axelrad Clinic has the following nutrient combination and dosage:

Vitamin A (as beta carotene) - 10000 IU
Vitamin E (as d-alpha tocopherol succinate) - 100 IU
Riboflavin (vitamin B2) - 25 mg
Zinc (as zinc picolinate) - 5 mg
Selenium (as selenomethionine) - 100 mcg
N-acetyl-l-cysteine (NAC) (free-form) - 100 mg
Milk thistle (silybum marianum) extract (seed) (standardized to contain 80% silymarin) - 100 mg
Mixed carotenoids (from lutein, lycopene and zeaxanthin) - 500 mcg

Generally, for the guys, I dose this one capsule in the AM and one at bedtime. However, it's fine to take 2 in the AM instead.

Sperm Support Supplement 3 - Ashwagandha + Rhodiola

The next supplement I give as a general male fertility enhancer contains Ashwagandha plus Rhodiola and is detailed in Chapter 12 under "Energy Reserve Replenishing Supplement 2".

283

It's a mix of "adaptogenic" herbs, and the two in this supplement that I believe are most helpful for male fertility are Ashwagandha and Rhodiola.

There are other plant-derived adaptogens in this formulation as well that support healthy mood and faster recovery from stress. So, it's a great (and very safe) supplement:

Sensoril®† Ashwagandha Root & Leaf Extract (Withania somnifera) - 250 mg
Rhodiola Rosea Root Extract (Rhodiola rosea) - 200 mg
Astragalus Root (Astragalus membranaceus) - 150 mg
Holy Basil Leaf (Ocimum sanctum) - 150 mg
Schisandra Berry (Schisandra chinensis) - 100 mg
Additional Foods & Extracts (Indian Gooseberry (Amla Fruit), Seaweed (Laminaria digitata and Ascophyllum nodosum)) - 145 mg

My generally recommended dose is two tablets in the morning.

Sperm Support Supplement 4 - L-Carnitine

L-Carnitine is, by far, one of the most studied nutritional compounds for male fertility.

It's an amino acid that is crucial fuel for the high-rate cellular metabolism required for both the creation of the sperm and their function as well (specifically in the area of motility).

Be a little careful with this one. It's generally well-tolerated even at substantial doses, but in some cases I've seen where it can be a little overstimulating.

We use 600mg capsules and our target dose for general male fertility support is 2 capsules twice daily (which adds up to 2400mg daily).

If you're doing this on your own, it's a good idea to start with 1 capsule twice daily at first, then about 7 days later increase to 2 capsules twice daily as indicated above.

(The exact supplements we use in clinic are listed in our online store, which you can access via our free portal **Axelrad Clinic Academy**. Visit https://axelradclinic.com/awaken to sign up.)

Common Questions And Answers

Will having intercourse too often cause my partner's counts to drop?

Yes, if you are having intercourse daily or twice daily then the counts will not be as high as if you've waited a few days.

However, if your partner doesn't have serious issues with sperm count, it's not something to worry about at all.

In fact, I believe that in many cases couples who aren't conceiving may not be having *enough* sex. While it's true that timing is important as far as ovulation, I believe that trying to be too exact with the timing can have the opposite of the intended effect, making intercourse mechanical and stressful.

My partner isn't interested in doing anything special. What should I do?

Focus on your own self-care 100%. Do your meditations, be consistent with self-directed loving-kindness, follow the eating and hydration strategies, and get your sleep.

I've found – both in my own life and when advising patients – that the best chance we have to change others is when we focus on changing ourselves.

I can't tell you how many cases I've had where, coming in, my patient was beside herself with frustration about her male partner's unwillingness to do anything in the realm of self-care.

And, in almost every case where that patient committed to their own self-care, letting go of what is impossible to control (someone else's behavior and choices), the male partner started to take note of the positive changes in their partner and, eventually, began to make changes of their own.

Part Four
Keeping Your Focus

"What the caterpillar calls the end, the rest of the world calls a
butterfly."
– Lao Tzu

Chapter 19 - You Don't Get A Special Trophy For Doing This Alone

It's a very tough thing when we're not getting something we want. It can be a real blow to our egos because, growing up, most of us got subliminal messages that people who don't achieve things are somehow losers or inferior in some way.

We're taught to think, "Maybe they're not so smart, or maybe they're lazy. Maybe they just don't have the education or the natural talent."

Whatever it is, when things don't end up in a good place for someone, the common tendency is for others to see it as a weakness, a deficiency, a flaw. Or, the person simply isn't trying hard enough.

Life is just competitive like that. I don't know why that is but for whatever reason there's a hard-wired need for us to feel valuable, loved, and important and, for whatever reason a lot of us take that to mean we must prove ourselves by exceeding others in some way.

So, when things aren't going well in the getting pregnant department, it is easy to fall into that same trap, thinking it is somehow a statement about your value, your worth, your importance.

I remember a patient of mine from the very early days of my practice, before I was a fertility specialist. She was suffering with breast cancer and was scheduled for a double mastectomy.

She was being treated at MD Anderson here in Houston, which attracts patients from all over the world due to its reputation as a top hospital for cancer.

She came to me mainly because she was only in town for a short time, had been doing acupuncture in her hometown and had found it to be relaxing for her.

I only worked with her a brief time. We did about 3 treatments prior to her surgery, then I visited her in the hospital a couple of times afterwards.

But, it was her visit the evening before her surgery I'll never forget.

I'd put the needles in and when I was about to leave the room, I told her, "While you're resting on the table, I want you to visualize tomorrow and that everything goes perfectly. The surgery is a complete success, the doctors do their job perfectly, and you are completely healed from the cancer."

I then left the room and let her rest for 25 minutes.

When I came back in the room she had tears running down her face. I asked her if she was OK.

"You're the first person who gave me permission to see this as a positive thing. Everyone else is criticizing me for this decision, saying things like it's too extreme and I'm letting them 'violate' my body or 'take away my femininity'. I was just realizing as I did your visualization that it was the first time I truly opened up and let myself feel good about my decision."

So, I asked her, "Well, those people saying those things, have any of them ever had cancer?"

"No," she answered.

Honestly, I take a couple of deep breaths to keep myself from becoming too angry when I hear people who spout fear and judgment about treatment options for diseases or issues they've never had.

Like people who rail against antidepressants who've never been clinically depressed.

Or, people who say immunosuppressant therapy is wrong who've never had severe autoimmune disease to the point where they were almost dead or severely disabled.

Or, people who say IVF is a cop-out or toxic or extreme - yet they've never had to deal with any fertility issues themselves.

Of course, in their minds, they'd "accept their fate" and be OK with it if they *did* have those issues. And, maybe some of them would do that.

But, faced with a real situation where *they* were the ones who were severely ill or being denied their dream of having a baby, I'd like to see what they do.

This isn't a game, it's not a race, and nobody's getting points for doing it a certain way vs. another way.

It's simply a choice. YOUR choice and yours ALONE.

And, this isn't like other things in terms of achievement. To get to a certain position in your company, or to have a certain social or financial status takes external effort and - to a certain extent - "luck".

In that world, there are tangible rewards for hard work, for focus, for staying on track and reaching your goals.

290

But, the thing is that in this case - where you're trying to have a baby - nobody's going to give you a trophy for doing it all yourself. You're not going to get any special status or reward for not taking medication or not doing IVF.

In the end, you're either going to have a child or you're not. That's pretty much it.

Now, I understand there are some people who for their own moral and ethical reasons simply will never choose to use assisted reproductive techniques like IUI, IVF, or even basic fertility medications.

I totally respect everyone's right to choose their path.

But, I see a lot of people who hold themselves back from moving forward with getting help - not because of a religious or moral belief - but simply out of shame, guilt, or fear of how they'll be perceived if they can't "do it on their own".

Or, they've heard so much negative and fearful talk about the process that they are terrified to even start.

First off, there is no shame in getting help and there's no shame in taking medication. Neither of these situations makes you less strong, less worthy, less of a shining, brilliant light than you already are..

Secondly, for the vast majority of people who undergo it, the IVF process - from what I've personally witnessed - is *not* the horrible dark experience so many make it out to be.

Can it be stressful? Of course. Are the injections and procedures less than ideal in many aspects? Absolutely.

But, if you go into it with the right mindset, ready to do what you must do to get where you want to go, you can do it without losing your mind or your dignity.

I've seen so, so many couples who - for whatever reason - struggled and struggled and struggled on their own for several years and, when they finally let go and did IVF, they responded like the most fertile couple on Earth. The embryos produced were extremely healthy, the pregnancies healthy, the babies healthy.

I understand everyone must come to terms with this in their own time. But, at the same time I think that if you take all the judgment, guilt, and shame away and just look at IVF for what it is - a little human assistance for nature - it is no longer the monster it seems to be.

IVF Is Not "Unnatural" – It Facilitates What Nature Already Knows

People say IVF isn't "natural". Well, I challenge those people to prove to me how it isn't.

True, there are some medications involved that push the ovaries a little harder than they normally would be.

True, in most cases these days they use ICSI (Intracytoplasmic sperm injection - where they inject a sperm into the egg), which removes the element of egg and sperm choosing each other.

True, the embryos incubate outside the mother's body for 5 days or so and are sometimes frozen for later thaw and transfer.

But, how is nature still not doing everything?

Nature is making the eggs, nature is making the sperm, and it is nature that sparks the fertilization process and begin to shape the embryo…

Nature is also building the lining and opening the receptive channel for implantation.

Nature is doing all of it.

Sure, it's getting a little help. But, that's it.

In fact, I'm going to say that when IVF doesn't work it's not because "the IVF failed". It's because for some reason nature couldn't successfully complete its life-creation process.

In my experience, having helped so many couples have babies with and without IVF, I no longer see any difference. There is about a 10-day window where the woman is injecting extra FSH and LH. There is another 5-day window where the embryo is incubating.

And, the rest is just like any other pregnancy.

ISCI Is Not Going Against Nature

Here's something else I want you to consider.

If I take a seed, go outside, and plant it in the ground in a place and time of my choosing, is that going against nature?

I guess if you're an absolute purist, who would prefer that we all still lived in caves as hunter-gatherers, it is. You'd say humans should never plant anything manually, we should just let the seeds scatter with the wind and let the plants grow where nature puts them.

There's nothing wrong with that view, either. I respect it.

But, I simply don't see the intentional planting of a seed as a sign of weakness, or of extreme manipulation of nature.

This goes for IVF itself as well as ICSI - which is also controversial.

There are many who, in my opinion, spread unnecessary and unwarranted fear about ICSI. That it is a form of "assault" on the egg and nature itself.

I couldn't disagree more, and I believe these kinds of extreme beliefs do a HUGE disservice to couples considering IVF by encouraging shame and guilt around the process.

Nature is more resilient and intelligent that you can ever imagine. Yes, it is intricate and delicate at the same time, but I truly believe - based on what I have seen over the past decade - that IVF, ICSI, and related procedures are valid, safe, and viable tools to facilitate conception.

Don't Let Others Control Your Narrative – Make Decisions That Align With Your Goals And Desires

I don't have a specific agenda for you to do IVF, IUI, or any other fertility treatment. Honestly, as crazy as this sounds after you've read this entire book, I don't even have an agenda for you to have a baby at all.

My agenda is simply this - to help you get to a place where you are making empowered, informed, and free choices for yourself.

Everything in this book is a choice. It's something YOU must commit to of your own free will and make happen - because nobody's coming to bail you out or "fix" this.

As I said above, even if you do choose IVF to help you conceive, nature is still going to have to be strong enough to finish the job. And, it is up to YOU and you alone to ensure that strength is there, within you, when the time comes.

Whatever you choose, I support you completely, as long as you aren't choosing to intentionally hurt yourself or anyone else. If you are choosing to love yourself and, through that love, increase your connection to your dreams and your destiny, it doesn't matter to me ONE BIT what your choice is.

Just make sure you know that if you are struggling with guilt, shame, or fear over the decision whether to get help via conventional or other means - the only one judging you, shaming you, or making you feel guilty is you.

You can make a different choice.

Chapter 20 - It's Not Fair And Why That's A Good Thing

Now I want to speak specifically to women who are married to men. So, if that's not you, you can probably skip this chapter.

I've seen relationships come apart around babies. Whether the babies end up coming or not, the journey to parenthood can be a true test of the bond between married couples.

One thing that's important to say up front here is that, as a woman, you don't need a man to have a baby. You never did, and you never will.

True, you need sperm and hence, all things being equal, you would need to have intercourse at least once to get pregnant. But, after that, it's all you.

That's the immense power you possess.

Now, I don't want to get into a discussion about the role of men in the family, the psychology of growing up without a father figure, and other such things. It's a very deep subject that probably requires an entire book in itself.

The reason I'm pointing this out - your unique ability to produce a tiny human being with nothing more than a few decent sperm and a relatively healthy egg - is because I want you to own this power completely.

In other words: Make this process *yours* first, then make it "ours".

I see a lot of women who spend what I feel is an inordinate amount of time focusing on what their husband is or isn't doing regarding improving the situation.

Maybe your husband's diet is terrible. Maybe he works too much or doesn't get his sleep or never drinks water or complains about taking one multivitamin a day much less a few extra supplements to ensure his side of the equation is as healthy as possible.

Maybe you have a husband that is super-supportive and on board and engaged which is awesome, too.

But I still want you to read this because it's important.

Regardless of whether you have moral support, whether you're 100% on the same page with your spouse or not, whether it seems like he even wants a baby or not…

If you want this, that's all that matters in the end because - in the end - you will make the baby. You - and only you - will be MOTHER.

Focus on yourself and prepare your body to be the vessel for one of the greatest miracles anyone can ever be part of. Do the things recommended in this book and don't wait for anyone - including your husband - to be on board.

I remember when I was going to have my first child. I was terrified. I knew my life was about to change forever and, honestly, part of me felt like running away as far as I could.

Then, I met my baby. And, my heart melted, and everything changed. Everything.

You are simply in a different position than your male partner. He'll never be able to relate to the kind of bond you desire and will have with the baby you carry or even the one you adopt, if that's what ends up happening.

It's just different, and it's meant to be that way.

I'm telling you this because I've seen a lot of what I feel is unnecessary and unproductive heartache in many of my patients who spend a LOT of time focusing on trying to recruit a stubborn husband into their process of preparing for baby.

I'm not saying it's bad to *want* more support, more empathy, more encouragement. And, obviously it's up to you how important it is for you and what you're willing to tolerate in your marriage.

What I'm simply saying is that the more you focus on you - on loving yourself, supporting yourself, nourishing and nurturing yourself - the more you will be creating the conditions that open the gate into motherhood for you.

So, don't wait for anyone's approval or for anyone to go along with you on the journey of transformation this book represents.

Transform yourself, and through that you will effortlessly transform everything else. I promise.

Yes, we have treatment options for people outside the Houston area to help you optimize your egg quality and get pregnant as soon as possible.

Visit https://axelradclinic.com/remote for details and availability.

Chapter 21 - How To Keep Going When It Seems Like Nothing Is Working

"The struggle is REAL." Heard that before?

It certainly can feel that way. The pressure, the anxiety, the constant obsessive thoughts around baby, baby, baby.

I want you to realize a couple of things...
1. The situation you find yourself in is temporary. Regardless of the outcome, it will pass.
2. It is not mandatory for it to feel like a struggle.

Earlier in the book, we went over my Transforming Stress Into Fertility process, where you learn to shift your emotional state at will, so you can lessen the tension and overwhelm that comes from focusing on tense, anxious feelings.

Sometimes, though, even that doesn't seem like enough. Sometimes, the wave just swells and carries you off.

The Deeply Medicinal Power Of Gratitude

It is impossible to be in a state of fear, anxiety, anger or frustration while expressing deep, sincere gratitude.

Gratitude is a state of acknowledging abundance and the love of others around us. This abundance and love are a natural extension of the love and abundance the Universe is continually expressing towards us each moment.

By saying "Thank You" we open the door for that Universal Love to enter our lives and hearts. And, when it does, our bodies respond by relaxing and becoming more peaceful.

The physiology of a relaxed state promotes tissue healing and healthy circulation and reduces inflammation. It encourages emotional calm and clear thought.

Cortisol and adrenaline -- the dominant hormones of fear -- are shifted into a lower gear as endorphin and serotonin -- the dominant hormones of pleasure and contentment -- are shifted upwards.

Blood vessels relax. Brain activity shifts from limbic "fight or flight" dominance to the more calm, clear centers of reason. Right and left brain fall into deeper synchrony, amplifying creativity.

Digestive organs function at a higher level which leads to increased nutrient assimilation.

The liver is no longer being bombarded with the toxins of increased oxidative stress associated with sad, angry, anxious emotional states. It is better able to do its job managing the body's hormones and neurotransmitters and detoxifying the blood.

(And, as we've learned from the earlier parts of this book, all of those shifts are immensely helpful to your eggs and the neuroendocrine flow that leads to conception and full-term pregnancy.)

You see, "Thank You" is a phrase that, when said with sincerity and purpose, reverberates into the body's healing system and awakens its profound power.

So, when you find yourself being overcome by that wave of sorrow or anxiety or anger... First things first, acknowledge it and love yourself anyway.

Then, take a moment to truly reflect on the blessings in your life -- the simple ones especially. For each one, inwardly say "Thank You" and fill your heart with a deep sense of sincere gratitude.

This is profound medicine.

The "Five Daily Gratitudes"

A simple practice I've learned to do - and have made a daily habit - is to simply think of 5 things I'm grateful for every day.

I do this as I'm going to sleep. Eyes are closed, and I just take a minute to say "Thank You" for five things in my life.

- Could be a person and the things they do for me, or teach me, or the ways in which they challenge me, or the opportunities they present for me to live my purpose.
- Could be things I have that make my life easier, more meaningful, more prosperous.
- Could also be problems and challenges I'm facing that are helping me grow stronger and gain more wisdom.

Sometimes, I'm grateful for the day being over. We all have days like that.

Whatever it is, I just do my best to say "Thank You" with sincerity and an open heart.

I'd advise you to make this a daily habit, too. But, even if you're not doing this every day, it is a powerful way to navigate through the storms that sometimes arise on the seas of life's journey.

(Our online community will keep you accountable and engaged in your Five Daily Gratitudes and the other self-care rituals of

Awakening The Seed. Visit https://axelradclinic.com/awaken to learn more on joining.)

Chapter 22 - Some Final Words Of Hope And Encouragement To Keep You Going

I've worked with thousands of women and couples along their family-building journey. And, just like with anything else, sometimes people don't end up exactly where they thought they wanted to be.

In each case where a biological child seemed out of reach, there was a very natural "pivot" that occurred where the decision was easy and natural.

When I look back on my life - and I'm certain you can say the same - there have been many difficult decisions along the way, where I had to step outside my comfort zone and just move forward even though I wasn't "sure" what the outcome would be.

(Can we ever be "sure"? That's a deeper question for another book. ;-)).

Yet, if I think back to those moments when I reached the decision point, I did have certainty that it was time to make the decision, even if there was no way to know the outcome.

In other words, I knew I was making the *right* decision for me.

And, in each one of those cases, the magical "pivot" occurred when I finally did a very critical thing that you will also do if/when the time comes...

I made the decision when I finally let go of the outcome.

Notice I didn't say "let go of wanting the outcome". That's an important distinction, especially in cases such as these where we're

303

finding ourselves in the middle of what can feel like a deep, existential crisis.

There's a peace that instantly settles over me when - faced with a seemingly difficult decision - I reach a point where I'm ready to move forward and accept defeat if that's what comes out of it.

Avoiding failure is a lot harder - and takes a lot more energy - than pursuing success. There's so much fear wrapped up in avoiding things.

We talked earlier in the book about the energy it takes to swim against the current vs using the pre-existing flow to take you where you want to go. In that case, we were talking about harnessing Nature to help you achieve your goal of conception and pregnancy a lot faster than you can on your own with raw effort.

It takes a lot of energy and creates a lot of strife to keep "pushing away" things we don't want. So much so that, in the end, we often end up "burning out" before we even get close to our desired destination.

If you've read this far... You're getting a special prize because this is one of the great secrets of achievement in general - and it works even more powerfully in the realm of fertility.

Honestly, if I could get away with it I'd tell every single patient who walks in my clinic, "We're going to start by giving up. Just surrender your need to have a baby, right now. And, let's focus all our energy and time on making every moment one of joy, gratitude, and purpose. The rest will take care of itself."

Problem is... most people can't hear that. They aren't in a place to process that.

What they hear is that annoying AF thing that everyone else says to them, "Oh… just stop trying, stop thinking about it, stop making such a big deal out of it and it will happen."

That is not what I'm saying… at all.

When I say, "give up" and "surrender", I don't mean "stop wanting it" or "stop trying". I mean, "Let go of the outcome and focus on the day-to-day things that give you strength."

Put even more succinctly…

"Fall in love with the process."

Allow yourself to become immersed in loving yourself, caring for yourself, breathing your Embryonic Breath and doing your Five Daily Gratitudes. Drinking your water and relishing your rest and sleep.

Just surrender to the moment. Be present. Yes, you want a baby and a part of you always will regardless of the outcome. Let that desire be your calling into a life of greater purpose and meaning right now.

By doing this now, you will set the stage to be ready for whatever is to come. I'm betting on you and I believe in you 100%. If you really invest yourself in the process outlined in this book, I'm betting on you to reach that "crossover point" into conception and pregnancy.

Which brings us back to the topic of this chapter which is how to know when it's time to move on.

"Moving on" is another "crossover point" and if you ever do reach it, you'll just *know*. Trust me on that.

In the meantime,… Immerse yourself in loving-kindness, mercy, and gratitude. Feed yourself with nature's most essential elements: Water, proteins and fats, regular and restful sleep, and a profound sense of wonder at this miracle we call "life".

That pretty much wraps it up for this book. I want to congratulate you on finishing. The fact you're reading this is, in and of itself, an indicator of your commitment to live a happy, fulfilling, purposeful life.

I wish you all that and more. And, I trust that you will discover just how beautiful you are… A true light like no other, right here, right now.

With love and gratitude,
Chris Axelrad, M.S.O.M., L.Ac., FABORM
Founder and Director of The Axelrad Clinic
https://www.axelradclinic.com

P.S. I really hope you enjoyed this book. If so, it would be super-helpful to me if you took just a few minutes to write a quick review here: https://axelradclinic.com/awaken-reviews. *Thank you in advance for spreading the word to help others on their journey to start or grow their family.* <3

And… don't forget. You're always welcome to attend one of our remote treatment intensives or take advantage of other remote support options. Just visit https://axelradclinic.com/remote for details on that.

Appendix

"Be careful what you water your dreams with. Water them with worry and fear and you will produce weeds that choke the life from your dream. Water them with optimism and solutions and you will cultivate success. Always be on the lookout for ways to turn a problem into an opportunity for success. Always be on the lookout for ways to nurture your dream." - Lao Tzu

Appendix 1 - Why Chinese Medicine Helps So Much – And How To Find The Right Practitioner

When I attended my graduate studies program in Chinese Medicine (which is a rigorous 4-year program, BTW), I was mainly interested in the herbal and meditative aspects of the art.

I'd heard of acupuncture but had never tried it myself.

In Texas, where I live, in order to attain a license we must study not only all the fundamentals of Western Medicine including Anatomy, Physiology, Pathology, Pharmacology, Microbiology, and more, we must also learn the entire system of Chinese Medicine including the physiology, etiology, diagnosis and treatment of disease with Acupuncture (over 300 points), Herbal Therapy (over 300 individual herbs and 200+ formulae), Food Therapy, and a range of other techniques including medical massage, cupping, and heat therapy.

Acupuncture fascinates me. When I first encountered it at the American College of Acupuncture and Oriental Medicine (where I began my studies in 1999) I was, to be perfectly honest, skeptical about it.

Again, I'd entered the college much more interested in the herbal lineage which made more sense to me coming from a Western background.

As I observed more and more cases in the school clinic and even underwent a few treatments myself, skepticism quickly turned to wonder.

One personal experience in particular solidified my understanding that, indeed, with acupuncture we have something very powerful even if we still can't completely map out how it works.

As a quick aside... The reality is much of medicine, including conventional medicine, is based purely on what we call "empirical" evidence. Meaning, "we're not sure how it works, we just know it works".

Areas of modern medicine where the mechanisms are poorly understood yet the effectiveness and the art are unquestioned include anesthesia, antidepressants, and many others.

Look up a well-known medication, and when you pull up the pharmacology section (this is where all the scientific jibber-jabber lives) you will more than likely find a sentence at the beginning that goes something like this:

"The precise mechanism of action of [main compound in drug] as a [drug class] is unknown, but its effect is believed to result from [a theoretical idea about how the drug works]."

In the case of eszopiclone, which is the molecular name of the oft-prescribed sleep medication Lunesta^{tm}, that sentence reads:

*The precise mechanism of action of **eszopiclone** as a **hypnotic** is unknown, but its effect is believed to result from **its interaction with GABA-receptor complexes at binding domains located close to or allosterically coupled to benzodiazepine receptors**.*

What they're basically saying is, "We don't know exactly how it works, but here's a plausible theory based on other scientific theories that we believe are true."

Kind of interesting, right?

What this means is that, for most pharmaceutical drugs, nobody really knows for sure how they work, we just know they work.

So, back to my interesting acupuncture experience when I was a first-year student at the college.

I used to suffer from fairly severe seasonal allergies, what we call "hay fever" down here in the southern United States.

The congestion, sneezing, eye irritation, and other symptoms were often so severe as to be unbearable and hardly responded to over-the-counter antihistamines and decongestants.

As a student at the school I was entitled to free acupuncture treatment in the clinic during any clinic shift. I thought, "Heck, let's go see if I can get this hay fever worked on."

I walked into the clinic, filled out the paperwork, and shortly thereafter I was in a treatment room with 2 student interns and a teacher-supervisor discussing my case.

After they decided what they were going to do, I got up on the treatment table and the interns started placing needles. I remember they selected two points down on my lower leg, a point on the palm of my hand just below my thumb (I'd be lying if I said that one didn't sting a little bit for a second), and a point on my ear.

Yep. My ear. That was a whole new thing to me at that point.

Then they told me to just rest for a little while and left the room.

What happened next I'll never forget.

After about five minutes of just lying there resting, I suddenly felt a gentle "rushing" sensation all around my nose and inside my sinuses as the fluid and pressure just started draining out.

My nose wasn't running or anything like that. No discharge at all.

The best way I can describe it is my sinuses felt like a water balloon and suddenly someone had made a little hole in it and the water was just slowly, steadily draining out.

Five or so minutes later I was completely clear. I was breathing normally. Zero sinus pressure. All the itchiness in my eyes was gone.

Just like that.

Over the next several days I thought about this "strange" (at that time, anyway) occurrence. I'd never experienced anything like this before.

Growing up in a very Western, very conventional household, I was plagued by the same obsession with explaining everything as everyone else.

And, it was about a week or so later that a very clear, rational, and plausible explanation did come to mind.

"Maybe the needles somehow triggered my body's natural antihistamine and anti-inflammatory system into action – kind of like turning up the volume on my body's innate process."

And to this very day, that's still how I explain acupuncture's mysterious – yet incredible – power to facilitate change and movement in the body.

You'll find about as many theories on how acupuncture works as you'll find scientists.

To this day if you ask me, "So, how does acupuncture help with fertility?" my initial answer is exactly this:

1) Acupuncture changes circulation to bring more blood into the pelvic organs, including the ovaries and uterus, so they receive more nutrients and clearer signals from the brain, and are more easily flushed of metabolic byproducts (i.e. oxidative chemicals, etc.).

2) Acupuncture calms the neuroendocrine system (the connection between the Central Nervous System and the endocrine system) so that there is less interference – which is a big thing when we're trying to optimize how the central hormones FSH and LH are signaling the ovaries, and how the feedback from the ovaries is being processed by the brain.

3) Acupuncture shifts the body away from a chronic pro-inflammatory state and encourages tissue healing which leads to a more ideal environment for all body process including the maturation of the egg.

4) Acupuncture produces a profound sense of relaxation, even a mild sense of euphoria - as it stimulates a flood of endorphin release – and this helps a lot to counteract anxiety and low mood.

Are all the above effects of acupuncture scientifically proven?

Actually, yes. They are.

Acupuncture has been demonstrated in studies – both human and animal studies – to lead to circulatory, neuroendocrine, inflammatory, and mood changes.

But, as with the pharmaceutical drug I mentioned earlier…

The precise mechanism of action of **acupuncture needles placed at certain points on the body** *as a* **[circulatory | neuroendocrine | inflammatory | mood] modulator** *is unknown, but its effect is believed to result from* **[insert here any one of several prevailing theories on how acupuncture might work]**.

So, anyway, my point is simply this.

Acupuncture is capable of doing things in the body that are incredibly helpful for ALL types of chronic conditions INCLUDING infertility.

Acupuncture also has a role in acute care, in my opinion. Acute care is essentially emergency care. As you saw in the story of my personal experience with acupuncture, it is capable of producing rapid changes in the body.

I could tell you a great story about when a loved one of mine was in the hospital with severe hypertension they were not able to control with medication and how, after I inserted 5 needles at specific points within 10 minutes his blood pressure dropped from 210 over 140 to 117 over 76.

But I don't want to get too far off track.

(Also, just for the record, this family member is himself a physician, and he asked me to come treat him, so the attending physician went along with it and OK'd it.)

Skill And Experience Are Important

Just like with any other thing, the skill of the practitioner is very important in terms of the potential for a positive outcome.

Acupuncture needles are just needles. They don't do anything on their own. Kind of like a tennis racket is just a tennis racket. It doesn't play tennis on its own.

If I pick up that tennis racket to hit a few tennis balls, you might want to duck. Seriously.

But, if Serena Williams happens to be hanging around and I hand her the tennis racket. WOW. Power, accuracy, and amazingness are sure to ensue.

So, when selecting an acupuncturist to help with your fertility, I'm a firm believer that, whenever possible, you are best served (no pun intended) by selecting someone who has a special interest in fertility, if not an outright fertility specialist.

The acupuncture profession in the Western world has not yet reached the point where we have a lot of specialty practitioners, although that is rapidly changing.

When I graduated in 2004, there were no post-graduate doctoral programs at all, much less post-graduate doctoral programs with specialty focus.

Today, we have many post-graduate programs that focus in areas like gynecology, fertility, orthopedics, internal medicine, obstetrics, and others.

Early on in my practice (as I mentioned in the introduction to the book), I gravitated towards gynecology, endocrinology, and fertility. It was an obsession for me.

And not only was this emphasized on my website and in all my marketing materials, it was absolutely the emphasis of all the coursework I did after graduation.

To me, anyway, it's important to work with a practitioner who is fluent in the language of fertility, including the Western side, so you know you are in the hands of someone who is capable of spotting situations that require referral for additional testing and possibly more aggressive approaches than what we are able to offer as a standalone treatment.

I see all my patients as my sisters (and I do have a few brothers as well ☺) and when they ask me for opinions and advice I always come from the place of "what would I tell my sister to do?".

If my own sister was having fertility challenges and asked me what to do, here's what I would tell her.

First and foremost, seek out a fertility specialist MD to run all the requisite tests. Not that an OB/Gyn can't order the tests and do a good job interpreting them. They can. And if you live in an area where there aren't fertility specialists, then definitely start with your OB/Gyn.

Just keep in mind that a fertility specialist deals with fertility patients every single day. They are seeing all the different scenarios all the time. They will know what to look for and (generally speaking) will spot problems that an OB/Gyn may dismiss as irrelevant or miss altogether.

I would tell her for sure to also find an acupuncturist who specializes in fertility and begin the work of uncovering any less obvious (but potentially just as powerful) blocks that an MD fertility specialist likely won't pay attention to – which is basically everything I already went over in this book.

I would NOT tell her to just find "an acupuncturist" and "get acupuncture".

Again… that would be like saying "find anyone who can swing a tennis racket and enter them into the US Open."

Seriously, this baby/fertility thing is as important to you as winning the US Open is to a professional tennis player.

You want to find Screna Williams or Rafael Nadal if you can. Don't settle for an amateur.

How Can I Tell If An Acupuncturist Is Good At Fertility?

There's no "one-size-fits-all" answer to this question. But, here's a few things you can look for:

Fertility Acupuncturist Criteria #1 – Reputation

NOTHING, and I mean NOTHING trumps reputation. If you've heard from one or more people you trust (friend, doctor, colleague, loved one) about an acupuncturist who is known for helping a lot of people have babies, go to that acupuncturist and see if it's a good match.

Fertility Acupuncturist Criteria #2 – Certification

As of this writing, there is only one specialty board on Earth that certifies bonafide specialists in fertility, and that is The American Board of Oriental Reproductive Medicine (ABORM).

I had the honor of serving on the Executive Board for this organization over a 4-year period between 2012 and 2016, the last 2 of which I was President.

ABORM administers a yearly exam for practitioners who wish to become "fellows". The exam covers all of the Traditional Chinese Medicine knowledge around fertility AND is very thorough in its coverage of the fundamentals of Western reproductive medicine as well.

It's a serious exam. And, because I served on the board for 4 years and proctored several exams, I can tell you for a fact that people fail the exam every year.

Which is good because this way the exam ensures that only people who are serious about mastering the material can gain certification.

I can honestly say that the practitioners I met through ABORM are some of the most committed and conscientious I know.

So, if you have someone who is ABORM certified in your area (and you can easily find out here: https://aborm.org), by all means check them out to see if it's a good fit.

Fertility Acupuncturist Criteria #3 – Terminology

As you know, there's quite a bit of terminology around fertility.

Most of the patients I see have already done quite a bit of research on their own – or have been through some conventional treatments – before they land in my office.

That means they are likely familiar with a lot of the terminology of the "fertility world", like the names of medications, the standard acronyms (TTC, BFP, OPK...), and the hormones (FSH, AMH, etc.)

If you go for an initial visit with an acupuncturist who is promoting themselves as someone who treats infertility and they seem confused when you start using the standard terminology, this is not a good sign.

Again, if my sister came to me and said, "Yeah, when I said I was taking [insert common fertility medication name here] the acupuncturist didn't know what it was. Is that OK?"

Honestly (again, remember this is my *sister* we're talking about), I'd definitely say, "No, that's not OK."

Am I saying they wouldn't be able to help you? No, of course not.

I'm just saying if you live in an area where you can find an acupuncturist who "knows the ropes", definitely do that.

Fertility Acupuncturist Criteria #4 – Attitude

I'm sure a few of my colleagues will disagree with me on this one, but I feel like I must mention it.

If my sister came back to me and said her acupuncturist (or her OB/Gyn for that matter) told her fertility drugs were toxic, birth control pills were "the devil", that IVF was to be avoided at all costs, donor eggs were wrong (and I've heard ALL these and more from my patients) …

I'd tell her, "Run out of there. As fast as you can. And, find someone else."

Now, I'm not saying go find someone who's going to advocate IVF right away with no rationale as to why. Nor would I be comfortable with my sister seeing a doctor who just willy-nilly put her on any treatment without justification.

But, I truly believe that patients are best served when ALL options are on the table. Doesn't mean you use all the options. It simply means we're not coming at it with a pre-defined agenda.

The other thing to be wary of (again, this is in any case, not just with acupuncturists) is anyone who criticizes or tries to talk you out of your medical decisions.

Have I seen cases where a new patient of mine came in for help with their IVF cycle who I thought would likely get pregnant on their own if we just worked together for a few months?

Of course I have.

Would I ever tell that patient I think they should stop their IVF process?

Absolutely not. Never. Ever.

Why? Because I respect people's autonomy and I do not have a fixed agenda for people. And... the IVF just might work. Why would I play God?

Again... if my sister told me she'd decided to do IVF I would support her decision 100% and simply do my best to help ensure her IVF was successful.

So, any practitioner who claims to be a fertility specialist that brings shame or fear into the equation by telling my sister she's "wrong" or "shouldn't" choose a particular medication or procedure that is proven to work and is proven safe...

I would absolutely question that practitioner's judgment. And I believe it would be smart for you to question their judgment, too.

What About Chinese Herbs?

There's a reason I didn't really talk about Chinese Herbs in this book, even though it's an area of expertise for me.

In my experience Chinese herbal formulas are a lot more powerful than supplements and, as such, I strongly recommend you not self-prescribe them.

Plants, being living things, have a very powerful energy and very complex physiology.

What we call "medicinal herbs" are, for the most part, plants that don't taste so good yet have useful (and often powerful) effects on our bodies.

When we ingest herbs – especially when they're compounded into formulas – there is a "dialogue" that takes place. This "dialogue" is nature speaking to nature.

It's important to remember that we have been on this planet evolving along side plants for millions of years. This is a long-standing relationship that has developed over that time.

Taking the wrong herbs at the wrong times is, in my view, a lot more potentially problematic than taking the wrong vitamin at the wrong time.

For instance, unless you're under the supervision of a skilled herbalist (and in many states – Texas included – Acupuncturists are required to pass board exams in herbal medicine in order to receive a license) I would strongly advise against taking any herbal medications while taking hormones (i.e. during IVF stimulation or priming prior to a stim cycle).

Fact is, I have had many patients of mine take herbs both during the priming phase AND the stim phase of IVF (and even during pregnancy for that matter).

But, I'm doing so with a lot of specialized knowledge and experience.

I'm not trying to scare you here. I just want to impart a proper sense of respect for herbs as medicine.

Yes, they're typically safe. Yes, they're "natural".

And, no, that doesn't mean they can't do harm if used improperly.

So, whether you're trying naturally or with something like IVF, if you want to incorporate herbs I absolutely recommend you seek out a qualified, reputable, skilled herbalist to help you do it not only safely but effectively.

That's what I would tell my sister to do.

Use the same criteria to choose your practitioner as the ones I mentioned earlier. And… more often than not those guidelines will lead you to someone who is able to provide the acupuncture and herbal support in a skillful manner.

Yes, we have treatment options for people outside the Houston area to help you optimize your egg quality and get pregnant as soon as possible.

Visit https://axelradclinic.com/remote for details and availability.

Appendix 2 - In-Vitro Fertilization (IVF) Optimization - Special Supplement And Self-Care Rituals For Stimulation And Retrieval

IVF, in many ways, does present a special situation that needs to be discussed separately. But before we get into that discussion let's make something very clear.

As stated earlier in the book, IVF is not a substitute for nature. It merely facilitates something nature already does – namely FERTILIZATION.

In other words (again, as stated earlier in the book), while the physical act of fertilization of the egg by a sperm is facilitated, nature itself must do *everything* else.

- The follicle must respond to the hormones, secrete estrogens, and fill with fluid.
- The egg must grow in a way that keeps it both structurally and functionally sound.
- When the trigger shot is administered, the egg must undergo its final stage of maturation and including final separation of chromosomes to prepare for successful fertilization.
- After sperm is inserted into the egg, the nucleus of sperm and egg fuse into one, and the genetic material is prepared for the first cell division. At this point we have a new organism, a literal fusing of mother DNA and father DNA.
- From there, if the genetic material is wholly intact and energy is available to support them, billions upon billions of transformations occur until, roughly nine months later, a

completely-formed little human being is ready to come into the world.

At this point I want to say… If you are doing IVF and you skipped to this part of the book… STOP HERE and go back to read from the beginning.

Why? Because all that stuff I just mentioned… The REST of the book is what makes sure all that stuff has the best chance of happening as nature desires it to.

While some of the things I mention below may seem like a shortcut (and in certain cases MIGHT be enough on their own), the material preceding this chapter is absolutely the best way I know of to ensure the best possible outcome for you.

Optimizing Your IVF Outcome

When it comes to optimizing your IVF outcome, there are just two basic facts to consider:

1. Virtually all the drugs used for the purposes of stimulation are analogues or bioidentical versions of hormones your body already makes.

What this means is that the stimulation process is simply pushing nature to do more than it would on its own.

And, if you've been paying attention to everything I've been telling you in this book then you probably already know what I'm about to say…

Nature already knows how to do everything related to making a healthy egg and sperm, completing successful fertilization of the egg, growing the resulting embryo to where it is a fully-developed fetus with all the organs and tissues needed for survival outside the womb.

And that brings me straight to point #2.

2. Optimizing an IVF outcome is simply a matter of making sure nature has surplus energy and signal clarity so it can respond to that stimulation with power and precision.

Whether you're trying naturally or with IVF, the goal is always the same: Build as much reserve energy as possible, protect that energy, and ensure the "field" (aka your body) is as clear and calm as possible so the signals nature is sending can travel with minimal disturbance and turbulence.

If you've been doing all the stuff I told you up to this point, that's exactly what you've accomplished.

You've built a nice store of extra energy and really clarified the "field" where all these signals travel (aka the blood, nervous system, etc.).

That's why I say there's not that much difference between preparing for IVF or trying on your own. The same fundamentals apply.

With IVF the drugs are merely an amplified signal that pushes nature a little harder than it pushes itself... And the signal has the same message for the ovaries whether you're injecting it for IVF or allowing your body to do it on its own. And, that signal simply tells the ovaries to do what they already know and get those eggs ready to be fertilized.

Critical Differences Between Natural And Stimulated Cycles

Of course, there *is* a difference during a stimulated cycle as compared to a natural one. And, this difference is very important to consider which is why I'm even writing this chapter to begin with.

In order to make sure your IVF cycle goes as smoothly as possible with the absolute highest chance for healthy embryos and – ultimately, of course – a healthy baby, we need to consider a few things and make sure we're taking care of them.

1. Stimulation does cause biological stress

If you're someone who doesn't exercise other than normal daily activities like walking around, picking things up, getting in and out of the car or bus, and whatever physical movements are required by your job…

…and you decide you want to run a marathon…

…I'm going to guess you would not expect to just show up on the day of the marathon and run it without *any* preparation for the extra work your body was going to have to do in order to finish the marathon.

Running a marathon is beyond the norm of what your (and my) body does on its own. It's just not "natural" – although it is DO-able if one is prepared for it.

It is important to recognize that IVF stimulation pushes the ovaries past their normal everyday activity levels, in a similar way running a marathon does for the bones, muscles, heart, and lungs of the body.

So, one of the ways I prepare my patients for IVF is to make sure we prepare for the extra stress the ovaries (and, as you'll see, other body tissues) will undergo during the 10 or so days of the stimulation phase, plus any "priming" (hormones administered prior to the stimulation) that may happen in the days or weeks leading up to the start of stimulation.

Dietary Prep For IVF Success

Again, if you've been following my instructions in the book so far, you won't have to change much, if anything, about how you're eating.

The Sun Cycle Diet and my Simple Hydration Schedule have you covered in terms of ensuring the raw materials are there and the "field" of your body is as "interference-free" as possible.

However, it's important to point out that if you're going to be doing IVF make sure you eat your proteins and fats in the form of meat and eggs every single day.

(Again, if you are vegan or vegetarian who doesn't eat eggs, make sure you consult a trusted expert on these eating styles on how to ensure you have maximum protein and fat intake leading up to and during the IVF stimulation.)

So, really for IVF prep I strongly recommend you eat 2-3 eggs – with the yolks – every single day starting at a minimum 10 days prior to the start of your IVF stimulation medications.

Additionally, now is the time to cut out all beverages except straight water. No flavors, no juices, no teas, no glasses of milk... Nothing except water (and of course if you need that coffee or tea first thing in the morning, it's fine and if you like it with a little cream and sugar it's fine too, just don't overkill it).

326

Lifestyle Prep For IVF Success

Once again, you're well-prepared if you've been doing the stuff I have already taught you, especially the sleep routines, meditations, and exercises.

For IVF prep specifically, I cannot emphasize enough how important it is for you to get at least 8, if not 9-10 hours of sleep every night both before and during your stimulation phase.

Again, ideally this should be your norm by now. But, if for some reason you haven't been sleeping the recommended amount of time, make sure you start at least 10 days prior to your stimulation phase.

Acupuncture For IVF Success

I'm not saying this just because I'm an acupuncturist (although being an acupuncturist I'm a huge believer in it based on the powerful positive changes I see in the IVF patients I work with).

There is no "non-conventional" therapy that has been more closely scrutinized in terms of how it affects IVF outcomes than acupuncture. And, with good reason.

As with any intervention, you will find studies that indicate acupuncture positively affects success rates, and other studies that indicate it has no effect. There are even a few studies that claim acupuncture has a negative effect on outcomes.

If anything, to me what these studies tell us is that acupuncture is not "inert". It absolutely affects what the body is doing and how it is responding to the IVF process.

Where these effects come from is kind of mysterious because it is difficult to explain how a tiny needle inserted into a specific "trigger point" can influence egg quality and count.

What I always say when people ask me to explain how acupuncture can make such an impact on IVF outcomes is this:

1) Acupuncture – electro-acupuncture specifically – can be used very effectively to promote circulation to different areas of the body, including the ovaries and uterus via the uterine artery.

2) Acupuncture is a powerful trigger for endorphin secretion. "Endorphin" is a broad term referring to opiates the body itself makes. Not only are these powerful pain-reducing substances, they also induce deep relaxation and have calming effects on the Central Nervous System which, in turn, can lead to subtle changes in neuroendocrine function (how the brain regulates hormonal output, including FSH and LH).

3) Because acupuncture taps into this "neuroendocrine" circuit, a skilled acupuncturist can use the needles to elicit changes in just about every bodily system, from immune to metabolic to limbic to circulatory and beyond. That's because all these systems are internally regulated by different hormones and neurotransmitters.

The bottom line is that after treating thousands of people over the course of my career as an acupuncturist, I can say without any doubt that our bodies are capable of very rapid and significant changes when acupuncture is skillfully applied.

And, the changes are not "magic" nor are they "placebo". They are real changes initiated by an intelligent, self-regulating, incredibly precise system in response to a systematic, time-tested, very precise stimulus (the acupuncture needle).

And, when we repeat that stimulation on a weekly or twice-weekly basis over a period of weeks or months... the changes in how the body is innately functioning can have a huge impact on the outcome of an IVF (or natural) fertility cycle.

Remember... hormones are dosed in milligrams and micrograms. Even tiny amounts of hormone can have big effects.

And, on top of this, the amount of fluid inside a follicle is literally just a drop. So, the very thing that we most want to influence – the fluid that nourishes and protects the egg – is itself tiny.

At one time I was on the Executive Board of The American Board Of Oriental Reproductive Medicine (ABORM), where I served as President for 2 years from 2014 – 2016.

ABORM is a professional board that certifies acupuncturists as fertility specialists. The requirements to sit for the exam are serious, as is the exam itself. And, once an acupuncturist becomes a fellow of the board by passing the exam, we are required to recertify with fertility-specific continuing education on an annual basis.

I cannot recommend a better resource for finding a qualified acupuncture specialist in fertility. Just visit www.aborm.org where you can search for an ABORM-certified specialist.

Special Supplements for IVF Success

Here's where we get into some special cases in terms of supplements that I've found to be generally applicable for anyone doing IVF, regardless of "The Five Core Factors" from the previous chapters.

Just like a successful endurance athlete will "carb-load" (eat large amounts of carbohydrate) prior to an event such as a marathon, there are a few things IVF patients can ALL do to help with general needs during ovarian stimulation.

Special IVF Supplement 1 – A Wide Spectrum Antioxidant

We talked before about the fact that our cells burn energy and the burning of that energy generates a sort-of "cellular exhaust" that is comparable biologically to the exhaust in the air generated by a car burning gasoline.

In fact, when we talk about "oxidative stress" in biological terms, we're mostly talking about the stress caused from byproducts of normal cellular activities like growth, respiration, metabolism, production of chemicals, and other things cells do.

During IVF stimulation, because the ovaries are generating a lot more estrogen than they normally do (at safe levels, of course), many of the body's cells and tissues are working a little harder than normal – not only in producing the estrogen, but also in responding to it, deactivating it, and clearing it from the body.

All that extra activity is like pressing on the gas pedal of the cellular engine. It's going to rev up and run a little hotter than normal.

And, as a result, it's going to not only burn more fuel but generate more exhaust.

Taking a wide-spectrum antioxidant goes a LONG way to helping your body ensure that all this extra exhaust is handled as efficiently as possible to absolutely minimize the damage it might do to the eggs.

Again… oxidation is a normal part of what your body does. Absence of oxygen-burning processes in the body equals death. So, your eggs will be OK even though there are oxidative byproducts present.

What we don't want is excessive buildup of these oxidative byproducts because then we may be getting to where they damage the follicle and the egg inside.

The rituals and practices of this book are – to be honest – a masterclass on minimizing oxidative damage to your body, not just your eggs. You can use the practices in this book as a means of longevity, not just fertility enhancement (in case you haven't already figured that out).

So… you're welcome. ☺

But, again, during the IVF process we're going to absolutely be in a place where oxidative stress is increased because of all the extra work those cells are doing.

The wide-spectrum antioxidant is a great way to give us a little extra "insurance" against toxic buildup – on top of the already stellar practice of drinking water, getting plenty of rest, and staying as calm as possible (because angst and anxiety ALSO push on the "cellular gas pedal", burning energy that can otherwise be used to heal and cleanse).

The one we use at the clinic has following nutrient dose in ONE capsule:

Vitamin A (as beta carotene) - 10000 IU
Vitamin E (as d-alpha tocopherol succinate) - 100 IU
Riboflavin (vitamin B2) - 25 mg
Zinc (as zinc picolinate) - 5 mg

Selenium (as selenomethionine) - 100 mcg

N-acetyl-l-cysteine (NAC) (free-form) - 100 mg

Milk thistle (silybum marianum) extract (seed) (standardized to contain 80% silymarin) - 100 mg

Mixed carotenoids (from lutein, lycopene and zeaxanthin) - 500 mcg

And for most IVF patients we recommend 1 capsule in the morning and 1 capsule at bedtime.

Special IVF Supplement 2 – Royal Jelly

So, if energy is the name of the game with optimizing IVF, Royal Jelly is going to be a very important supplement for us to consider.

I like to think of the foods nature makes as a "language", in a sense. Certain foods are designed by nature to elicit a specific response in the parts of nature that consume that food… Just like certain words we say can certain different responses in the people who hear them.

Take fruit, for example. I believe it was mentioned earlier in the book, but if you think about fruit it is a summer food. It grows abundantly in the summer months (whether tropical or at more temperate latitudes). It's cool and refreshing and full of water. It has key minerals to replace those lost in sweat (after all, it's hot in the summer). And, it's high in sugar which, if we're on a long walk or working outside in the hot summer sun, will keep us going through the day.

Thinking of food this way, when we look at Royal Jelly, we've got some very interesting properties that make it perfect for the stimulation phase of an IVF cycle.

Royal Jelly is a sticky substance made by honey bees. The interesting thing about it, though, is that it is only consumed by the queen bee – hence the name "Royal Jelly".

The worker bees – and in a big hive there are tens of thousands of them – are busy literally round the clock collecting pollen, building and maintaining the nest, protecting the queen, and making honey which is used to feed the colony EXCEPT for the queen and the baby bees.

Once a larva is selected to be queen, it is exclusively fed "Royal Jelly" from that point forward for the rest of its life. It is the only bee that can consume the Royal Jelly in this manner as an adult.

The only other bees that are fed Royal Jelly are the baby bees for the first 3 days or so of their lives. After that, they consume honey like all the other bees.

The Royal Jelly, fed to the queen, is essentially a "super-food" that triggers the changes in her body that allow her to produce literally 1500 or so eggs every single day.

Royal Jelly, then, is designed by nature to convey massive amounts of energy and life-creating power to the queen bee, as well as a powerful shot of concentrated growth to baby bees during the first few days of life.

I've used it a lot in clinic. And, it never disappoints. It's a powerful nutrient but, more than that, I believe it conveys a message to our cells and tissues that is like the message it conveys to the queen bee – telling them to grow and multiply.

This makes Royal Jelly a very powerful substance for tissue growth and healing which, if you've been paying attention, is exactly what we want your eggs to do... We want them to GROW and STAY HEALTHY (i.e. continually heal themselves).

Now… I'm not saying you'll produce 1500 eggs by taking Royal Jelly. But, what I AM saying is based on my own clinical experience, it's a powerful superfood for IVF stimulation because it is such a dense, concentrated energy source and, in nature, it is used specifically for reproductive purposes.

In clinic we use Royal Jelly in powdered extract capsule form with a potency of 1500mg per capsule. The dose we use is 2 capsules every morning throughout the IVF process – both prep and stimulation phase.

Honestly, it's a very safe nutrient but there is one warning I must mention. **If you are allergic to bees do NOT take this supplement.** It can trigger a serious allergic reaction.

In all my time I've only seen this kind of allergic reaction occur once, so they are extremely rare. But still, I wanted to mention it.

Special IVF Supplement 3 – Ubiquinol (Micronized CoQ10)

We've mentioned this supplement before in Core Factor Three. And when it comes to IVF, there isn't a supplement that is more widely recommended than this one.

Ubiquinol is the micronized form of CoQ10. Really you can take either, but the thing with Ubiquinol is that, because it is more readily absorbed and utilized than CoQ10, you only need about 50% as much for the same effect.

Ubiquinol is rocket fuel for the mitochondria, which is why it's been so heavily studied as a supplement in IVF. One of the most critical components of a viable, healthy egg is an abundant population of healthy mitochondria, which are the "power plants" of cells.

As mentioned in an earlier chapter, once the egg is released from the follicle via ovulation (or retrieval), it must be able to – in large part - generate its own energy. And, the mitochondria are key to this.

So, the energy to get from 1 cell to 8 cells to blastocyst is going to depend heavily on the number and health of the mitochondria inside the egg at the time of ovulation.

That's why Ubiquinol is so important. Because it fuels the production and function of mitochondria it is essential if we're going to optimize your IVF outcome.

It's going to give your body the best possible chance of producing mitochondria in enough numbers and with enough energy producing capacity to support the cell divisions that take place during the first several days of embryonic life.

Another benefit of Ubiquinol is that it is an essential nutrient for blood vessel tissue repair. So, not only does it fuel the egg, it ensures the capillaries that carry oxygen and nutrients to the egg are as healthy as possible, too.

The Ubiquinol we use in clinic comes in 100mg gel caps and we typically recommend 100mg in the morning and 100mg at bedtime. Sometimes, depending on the situation, I might recommend 200mg twice daily instead.

Special IVF Supplement 4 – DHEA

For the warnings and general information on DHEA, refer to "Chapter 12 – Core Factor One: Abundant Energy Reserves". DHEA is a hormone and therefore needs to be treated differently than the other supplements recommended in this book.

One of the IVF cases I remember where DHEA made a big difference is a patient of mine who, after 4 days on stimulation drugs, was barely responding. Because she was on the max dose of stimulation meds things were not looking optimistic.

She'd been reluctant to take DHEA prior to this because of some things she'd read on the internet. At this point, though, she was willing to go along with my original advice which was to take 25mg of DHEA 3x a day.

She asked if it was too late, to which I replied, "I guess we'll find out. All I know is nothing's likely to change if you don't take it starting now."

So, she started that day and 48 hours later the response was night and day. Her estrogen started rising normally and… you guessed it… she went on to get pregnant and she now has a daughter.

Again, DHEA is a hormone. More precisely it is a "precursor" hormone for testosterone then estrogen. In other words, the body uses it as a building block along the pathway to making estrogen, kind of like rocks are used as raw material to make cement, or wood is used as raw material to make paper.

I would not recommend starting DHEA for the first time during a stim cycle without consulting your doctor first because if it isn't right for you it could lead to problems that would require stopping the cycle altogether.

So, start DHEA only if your doctor gives you the go ahead AND it is at least a month ahead of starting your stim cycle so there is plenty of time to discontinue it and return to baseline if you don't react well.

Signs of not reacting well to DHEA include nausea, headache, rash, diarrhea, increased blood pressure, and heart palpitations.

Increased acne and skin oiliness are not signs of an adverse reaction, necessarily. But, again… my best advice is get medical advice on this one rather than self-prescribe.

Typical dose in my clinic is 25mg morning, afternoon, and evening for a total of 75mg daily.

Common Questions And Answers

How long before my IVF stimulation should I start taking these?

As a rule, I'd say ideally at least 60 days before you start.

However, let me make something very clear.

I've had many, many cases of people who came to me for help with IVF – who were not taking any of these and were due to start their next cycle (after a failed cycle) in a matter of days – who had successful cycles taking these for just a few days prior to stimming.

Bottom line is, as I told that patient I mentioned who started DHEA mid-stims, "Nothing's likely to change if you don't start taking them now."

So… bottom line is just start taking them as soon as you can and don't worry if you're outside that 60-day window. I promise they'll still help a lot.

When should I stop them?

Typically, what I do is keep patients on them until we know there's a transfer scheduled.

If you've done IVF before or know someone who has, then you know that in many cases it might take 2 or 3 rounds of stimulation to get the desired result in terms of quantity and quality of embryos.

If a patient of mine does a retrieval then I will keep them on the IVF support supplements until they know whether they're going to do another one. This is typically after results are in, in terms of the number of blastocysts, how many blastocysts are normal (if PGD is being used), etc.

Is there a limit to how long I can be on them?

The doses I recommend are safe for long-term use so, no, there really is no limit except for DHEA.

Again, because DHEA is a hormone, it can accumulate in the bloodstream. So, if you're on DHEA and you've been taking it for more than a month or two, talk to your practitioner about it. In certain cases, I'll have my patients take a break from it. But this is on a case-by-case basis.

If you've done IVF before or know someone who has, then you know that in many cases it might take 2 or 3 rounds of stimulation to get the desired result in terms of quantity and quality of embryos.

If a patient of mine does a retrieval then I will keep them on the IVF support supplements until they know whether they're going to do another one. This is typically after results are in, in terms of the number of blastocysts, how many blastocysts are normal (if PGD is being used), etc.

Appendix 3 - Frozen Embryo Transfer (FET) Optimization - Special Supplement And Self-Care Rituals

Once the eggs are retrieved and fertilized, and we know a transfer is imminent (whether that is a fresh or frozen transfer), it is time to shift gears and prepare to receive the embryo.

It goes without saying, this is a very critical moment when the embryo is placed inside the uterus where, if everything goes according to "plan", it will burrow into the lining to begin – and eventually complete – the process of implantation or attaching to mother.

The process of implantation is largely a mystery. But, again, here's what we do know.

There's a lot of crosstalk going on between embryo and uterine lining during the initiation of implantation. And, for those signals to be clear and the process to unfold properly, the embryo must "hatch", and the lining must allow implantation to take place.

I say "allow" because, in essence, implantation is the only situation where a human body will intentionally allow a "not-self" organism to fuse with it and take nutrients from it.

Which, again, brings me to an important point. This allowing process is dependent on the mother's immune system being able to "turn itself down" so it doesn't block implantation from occurring.

There are a few key elements we must pay attention to at this time to make sure we give nature the best chance at successfully completing this phase which – again! – it already knows how to do.

1. We need a responsive lining that is full of nutrient-rich, well-oxygenated blood.

If you've been following my instructions throughout this book, we'll already pretty much be there. So, there's not really a whole lot more to do.

However, an embryo transfer is a precious moment... Especially in cases where there may only be one or two embryos to transfer after a long, long process. So, in a minute I'll share with you some of my best tips for ensuring your lining is as alive as it can be at the time of transfer.

Quick note here: You'll read all kinds of conflicting information about how thick the lining is "supposed" to be at transfer. Bottom line is the reason the information conflicts is because it can vary from person to person.

The most important thing is that the lining has three distinct layers – meaning it's "trilaminar" in the medical parlance. These three distinct layers are critical to how the lining functions and without them there is little to no chance of an embryo surviving.

In terms of actual thickness, I must say that I've never personally seen a transfer work when the lining was close to or less than 6mm. Not that I've even seen many transfers attempted at that thickness. But, the ones where it was attempted at this thickness – at least in the cases I've seen – did not work out in the long-term.

2. We want the lining to be soft and sticky.

What a lot of people don't know is that progesterone causes healthy lining to become spongy (soft) and sticky.

341

This is obviously a very smart thing nature is doing, then, as during a natural cycle the progesterone is in place for about 5 days prior to the arrival of the embryo.

It's like nature's way of "fluffing the pillow" if you will. Kind of a weird analogy but you get the point.

If the lining isn't soft enough – meaning there's not enough space and "give" for the embryo to burrow in – implantation might fail even though the embryo is healthy and the lining is, too.

And, if it's not sticky enough, well… it's not like the embryo is just going to "fall out" but all those secretions won't be there to help the embryo get a "foothold" as it begins the implantation process.

Things that negatively impact the structure and function of the lining

So, what would negatively impact the layering, softness, and stickiness of the lining? A few key things, at least in my estimation from doing this thousands of times.

First, and foremost, excessive chronic inflammation.

Now, again, I don't want you to worry because if you're following the steps I've already outlined throughout this book, you're already minimizing chronic inflammation.

But, if you're not doing those things, I'd strongly encourage you to go ahead and get started.

An inflamed lining will not have normal circulatory function – because no inflamed tissue has normal circulatory function. That's why it's called "inflammation" – there's all kinds of excess fluids and blood vessels in many cases are intentionally degraded around the site of injury to allow for more fluid and immune cells to enter the area, causing swelling.

Inflammatory states can also lead to thickening of the blood and, hence, potentially slow circulation and increase the tendency to form clots – neither of which are optimal for implantation.

We've already discussed how chronic inflammation arises in the body and we're already addressing it with our Three Foundations, Sun Cycle Diet, and other practices.

Second would be insufficient circulation into the lining.

Blood, as we discussed earlier, is a liquid tissue full of not only cells but information in the form of nutrients, chemical messengers called "cytokines", and (of course) hormones.

If the lining isn't receiving fresh blood on a continuous basis, it's not going to be getting the nutrition, hormones, and information it needs to grow and function properly.

On top of this, if the circulation isn't at least decent, old blood will not be removed efficiently so metabolic waste products may accumulate there.

Good news is – again – with everything I've taught you in this book – especially the hydration strategies and sleep rituals – you're already covering all the fundamentals to ensure healthy circulation into and throughout the uterine lining.

Last, but not least, would be lack of nutrients in the blood.

In order to construct healthy lining – which is a very delicate and intricate web of glands and capillaries – there must be ample supply of proteins and fats for structure, and glucose for energy, along with all the minerals, vitamins, and cofactors the endometrial cells need to do their work.

If any of these are significantly depleted or deficient, there could be problems along the way of "building" the lining and/or the lining may not be able to function as nature intends it to.

This is why I emphasize protein and fat so much in my Sun Cycle Diet. The relatively high-protein diet provides a surplus of building blocks not only for the follicles and eggs, but the lining as well.

And, the fats are key in providing the energy needed in the form of glucose WITHOUT the disruptive effects of insulin surges and crashes resulting from straight consumption of starches and sugars.

Dietary Prep For Successful Embryo Transfer

This is the same as dietary prep for stimulation.

Again, if you've been following my instructions in the book so far, you won't have to change much, if anything, about how you're eating.

The Sun Cycle Diet and my Simple Hydration Schedule have you covered in terms of ensuring the raw materials are there and the "field" of your body is as "interference-free" as possible.

Again, it's important to point out that, in my clinical experience at least, make sure you eat your proteins and fats in the form of meat and eggs every single day.

(Again, if you are vegan or vegetarian who doesn't eat eggs, make sure you consult a trusted expert on these eating styles on how to ensure you have maximum protein and fat intake leading up to embryo transfer.)

The only difference for embryo transfer is you can back off on the eggs if you want (which might be great news in case you're sick of them by now).

And, again, now is the time to cut out all beverages except straight water. No flavors, no juices, no teas, no glasses of milk... Nothing except water.

And in the case of transfer, if you want to be completely on the safe side, really minimize your caffeine intake as much as possible and even avoid it altogether if you can. Not that caffeine will cause a failed transfer... It's just to be sure we're not introducing too much into the internal environment at this very critical time.

Lifestyle Prep For Successful Embryo Transfer

Once again, you're well-prepared if you've been doing the stuff I have already taught you, especially the sleep routines, meditations, and exercises.

And, again, I'm going to sound like a "broken record" (which you probably have never experienced but it basically means I'm repeating myself over and over to point of annoyance), I cannot emphasize enough how important it is for you to get at least 8, if not 9-10 hours of sleep every night especially before and during the "two week wait".

Again, ideally this should be your norm by now. But, if for some reason you haven't been sleeping the recommended amount of time, make sure you start now.

Acupuncture For Successful Embryo Transfer

For many of the same reasons acupuncture is helpful for the stimulation phase, it is also helpful for transfer.

In fact, most of the studies done on acupuncture focus specifically on how it affects the outcome of the transfer, not the entire cycle.

I've had more cases than I can count of people who had one or more failed frozen embryo transfers (FETs) who came to me for help and got pregnant on the very next FET after weekly acupuncture along with the supplement protocol I'm about to outline here.

Important note here: Every single one of my patients is given the guidelines on sleep, hydration, and other things I discuss throughout this book. And I can tell you without hesitation the ones who implement them – even if we only a have short time to prepare prior to the FET – always have better outcomes.

In my clinic we do once or twice-weekly treatments (depending on the patient's schedule) leading up to the week of transfer. We try to start those as soon as we can, so we get at least 4 weeks of treatments in prior to the patient starting the estrogen priming.

Then, we do a special a "pre-transfer" session the evening before the transfer (or the morning of the transfer, schedule permitting) followed by a "post-transfer" session 4 or 5 days later.

Also, we encourage our patients to rest at home for at least 2-3 days after their transfer. That means taking time off from the job, avoiding

346

heavy physical work such as housecleaning, vacuuming, standing at the sink or kitchen for long periods of time, yardwork, etc.

After the post-transfer session, we continue weekly sessions until our patients reach 12 weeks of pregnancy.

With this cadence of treatment, including pre- and post-transfer and the weekly sessions before and after, plus the home rest, the success rate of our patients with FET is well above 70%. So, we're not changing this anytime soon. ;-)

Where to find a qualified acupuncturist

At one time I was on the Executive Board of The American Board Of Oriental Reproductive Medicine (ABORM), where I served as President for 2 years from 2014 – 2016.

ABORM is a professional board that certifies acupuncturists as fertility specialists. The requirements to sit for the exam are serious, as is the exam itself. And, once an acupuncturist becomes a fellow of the board by passing the exam, we are required to recertify with fertility-specific continuing education on an annual basis.

I cannot recommend a better resource for finding a qualified acupuncture specialist in fertility. Just visit www.aborm.org where you can search for an ABORM-certified specialist.

If there isn't an ABORM-certified specialist near you, consult with your Reproductive Endocrinologist. Oftentimes they do know who the experienced fertility acupuncturists are in the area.

Special Supplements for Successful Embryo Transfer

I've used this specific supplement protocol in its basic form many hundreds of times for embryo transfers. All I know is, based on the success rates we see with our patients, we will be changing it anytime soon.

It's going to be a little different depending on whether you're doing a fresh or frozen transfer.

Obviously if you're doing a frozen transfer, you know well in advance and can do the entire protocol as outlined below. If it's a fresh transfer, skip the L-Arginine and do the other ones.

Also, if it's a fresh transfer, you can generally stop any supplements you were specifically taking for stimulation. Again, always consult with your practitioner (if you have one) before changing anything.

Special Embryo Transfer Supplement 1 – Ubiquinol

Ubiquinol is the micronized form of CoQ10. Really you can take either, but the thing with Ubiquinol is that, because it is more readily absorbed and utilized than CoQ10, you only need about 50% as much for the same effect.

In the case of embryo transfer, the aspect of Ubiquinol we are most interested in is its role as an essential nutrient for blood vessel growth and tissue repair.

Taking ubiquinol prior to transfer and through the 12 weeks of pregnancy ensures the intricate web of blood vessels and capillaries that carry oxygen and nutrients to the embryo and fetus are as healthy as possible.

Another thing that I think is grossly underappreciated is the fact that Ubiquinol is the most abundant nutrient in heart tissue because of its role in sustaining the energy of the mitochondria. Obviously the heart is continually expending energy. It's literally the only muscle in the body that never stops moving from the time we're just a 6-week fetus until the day we expire.

So... given this fact I truly believe that taking Ubiquinol also ensures the baby's heart can function optimally. And, last time I checked, that's kind of important.

For the purposes of early pregnancy lining support (including during transfer time), the dose we recommend is 100mg in the morning and 100mg at bedtime.

Special Embryo Transfer Supplement 2 – L-Arginine (Frozen Transfer Only)

Because one of our important things to do is ensure blood flows freely into the capillaries of the lining, we're going to use L-Arginine as a helper.

L-Arginine feeds the nitric-oxide system of the body. You don't have to know how that works, so don't go Google it. Just know this: Sildenafil (aka "Viagra") works by modulating the nitric-oxide system of the body so that blood flow to the man-parts is increased and as a result, erections not only are easier to attain but also last longer.

Some fertility doctors will prescribe vaginal insertion of sildenafil suppositories in cases where the lining isn't thickening to adequate levels.

What we're going to do is just make sure your body has enough Arginine to manage its own nitric-oxide system in a way that keeps blood flow smooth and open as possible so that, hopefully, you won't need to worry about lining problems.

The potency of our L-Arginine at The Axelrad Clinic is 700mg per capsule and typically I'll have patients take 1 capsule every morning and another at bedtime **only during estrogen priming**.

So, you'd start the L-Arginine when you start the estrogen phase of the transfer cycle (most of the time this means you're taking estrogen but sometimes you might be injecting medication or taking letrozole).

Then STOP the L-Arginine when you start the progesterone.

Special Embryo Transfer Supplement 3 – Systemic Proteolytic Enzymes

Of all the transfer supplements, this is one is magic.

You'll read online that bromelain – which is highly concentrated in pineapple core – increases implantation rates. While it's mostly anecdotal, I do believe this to be true. Why?

Well, we talked about the "softness" of the lining. In terms of body tissue and cells, systemic proteolytic enzymes, or enzymes that help the body break down proteins in blood and tissue (not to be confused with *digestive* enzymes which break down proteins in the intestine) are an important key to making sure tissues such as uterine lining are soft, moist, and pliable.

Not only this, but systemic proteolytic enzymes also help the body naturally break down clots without acting like blood thinners. So, in my estimation and from what I've seen, unnecessary or excessive clotting in the lining is greatly minimized.

Key thing here is that these enzymes typically do not cause excessive bleeding, especially at the doses we use in clinic. *HOWEVER, it is obviously important before you take these to make sure you don't have any genetic or other predispositions to abnormally long clotting times.*

Now, if you've ever eaten pineapple core you know this: It's horrible. Bitter, weird texture… just nasty.

Therefore, I have all my patients take these systemic enzymes in capsule form instead. They get the same (if not more) benefit as they would by eating pineapple core without the nasty.

Which means they're much more likely to stick to it and get results.

The one we use has the following composition per capsule, and we usually recommend patients take 1 capsule in the morning and one at bedtime:

Nattozimes (2000) FU) exo/endo proteases - 129 mg
Serrazimes (20,000 U) exo/endo proteases - 33 mg

Common Questions And Answers

Will these supplements hurt my baby?

I can say with 100% confidence that, no, they will not.

I've used these thousands of times and there have been no adverse effects on the fetus whatsoever.

Will they conflict with baby aspirin?

A lot of REs will have their patients take baby aspirin for its gentle anti-clotting effects.

In my clinical experience, all these supplements at these doses are perfectly safe to take along with baby aspirin and, again, in about

70% of the cases I've worked with where previous transfers failed WITH baby aspirin, the next transfer worked after adding these supplements plus the acupuncture with no adverse events.

What if I'm taking a blood thinner like lovenox or heparin?

The safest thing to do in this case is omit the systemic enzymes. The L-Arginine up until starting the progesterone, and the Ubiquinol through the first 12 weeks are OK to take with lovenox or heparin, in my experience.

If you are on these blood thinners, however, I strongly encourage you to consult with your RE about any supplements you're taking.

When do I stop them?

In the absence of blood thinners, my clinical experience says you can take both the Ubiquinol and systemic enzymes throughout pregnancy if you wish. However, again, this is a decision you should make in consultation with your RE and/or Obstetrician.

One Last Reminder...

Yes, we have treatment options for people outside the Houston area to help you optimize your egg quality and get pregnant as soon as possible.

Visit https://axelradclinic.com/remote for details and availability.

AND

Because you're reading this book, **you have FREE, lifetime access to the Axelrad Clinic Academy,** our exclusive patient reference library that contains all the resources mentioned in this book and more, including:

- Simplified meal plans.
- Meditations and guided visualization tracks.
- Exclusive cheat sheets and critical reference materials.
- A special supportive online community of others who have or are still walking the same journey as you.
- Videos and other exclusive content only available to

Sign up for free, no strings attached, at
https://axelradclinic.com/awaken.

Printed in Great Britain
by Amazon

59644079R00220